Nutrition Made Easy

Lorraine Kelly
with Anita Bean

Virgin BOOKS

Published by Virgin Books 2009

2 4 6 8 10 9 7 5 3 1

First published in Great Britain in 2009 by
Virgin Books
Random House, 20 Vauxhall Bridge Road,
London SW1V 2SA

www.virginbooks.com
www.rbooks.co.uk

Addresses for companies within The Random House Group Limited can be found at:
www.randomhouse.co.uk/offices.htm

The Random House Group Limited Reg. No. 954009

A CIP catalogue record for this book
is available from the British Library

ISBN 9780753515525

The Random House Group Limited supports The Forest Stewardship Council (FSC), the
leading international forest certification organisation. All our titles that are printed on
Greenpeace approved FSC certified paper carry the FSC logo.

Our paper procurement policy can be found at www.rbooks.co.uk/environment

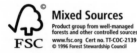

Mixed Sources
Product group from well-managed
forests and other controlled sources
www.fsc.org Cert no. TT-COC-2139
© 1996 Forest Stewardship Council
FSC

Typeset by Palimpsest Book Production Limited,
Grangemouth, Stirlingshire

Printed and bound in Great Britain by
CPI Mackays, Chatham ME5 8TD

Contents

Introduction

We have never had so much information available to us about what sort of food we should be eating to keep ourselves and our families healthy. The problem is that so much of it is contradictory and confusing, and we end up wondering exactly what we should be doing for the best.

We are told that red wine is good for us, but then warned about the dangers of overdoing the booze, especially at home when we tend to pour ourselves bigger measures than in the pub. Tea contains antioxidants, which can only be a good thing, but then we are lectured about the high levels of caffeine in our diet and drinking too much tea and coffee. Low-fat diet foods and drinks are often shockingly loaded with sugar and although food labels are a good idea they are often so confusing we are still in the dark as to just how good or bad certain foods are for us.

Maybe you are confused about how much protein and carbohydrates you need to eat, and exactly why we should all be having five portions of fruit and vegetables a day. And just what exactly constitutes a portion anyway? Then what about the salt content of our food? Why is too much salt so harmful and how can we cut down on our intake?

The danger of all this conflicting information is that we take it all with (forgive me) a pinch of salt and then ignore the really sound advice. It's a real minefield, but this book is here to help.

Let's get one thing straight – food is one of the great joys of life and should never be treated as 'the enemy'. What we all need to do is strike the right balance with what we are eating.

This book isn't about putting you or your family 'on a diet', because I happen to think that diets don't work. If you go 'on' a diet then inevitably you will have to come 'off' the diet and that leads to yo-yo weight loss, which is bad for your confidence, self-esteem and health.

This book is about giving you the information and the knowledge you need to have the healthiest possible eating plan: one that will last you for the rest of your life.

It is all too true that you are what you eat, and the food you consume can either make you happy and healthy or fat and miserable. Food can be used to make you feel calmer or more alert and can also increase your energy. The food you eat can help boost your immune system, help you have a good night's sleep and also provide comfort. If I feel under the weather, nothing helps more than a big mug of my mum's home-made chicken and vegetable soup. It is an instant pick-me-up.

We have to make sure we are eating a diet that

will help us live a long, healthy, happy life. When it comes to our children, it has never been more vital to ensure that we do the very best for them. We are teetering on the brink of an obesity epidemic. We have all seen fat babies in their pushchairs, overly plump young children and the teenage girls with their 'muffin tops' of excess flab hanging over their low-cut jeans. Unless there is a major change in eating habits, more than a quarter of the next generation are piling up horrific health problems for the future.

As parents we must take responsibility. We need to make sure our children are fed the right food as soon as they come off the breast and the bottle. They need to eat good wholesome grub and not be force-fed a diet of fast food and junk. I don't think it is realistic or desirable to ban them completely from eating sweets and crisps, but these foods should be looked upon as treats and not something to be guzzled every single day.

It is all about common sense and having the right information.

I really regret the way that what we used to know as 'Home Economics' does not have the importance or recognition it deserves in our schools. What could be more vital than knowing about what food to eat and how to cook it in the most effective and tasty way?

All of us need to take more care about what we eat and I think it is more important than ever to have a straightforward, no-nonsense guide to nutrition. We have written this book in a Q&A style – it means the vast subject of nutrition is broken down into more manageable chunks, making the whole thing, if you'll excuse the pun, easier to swallow. And, in addition to all the vital nutritional information, you'll find lots about the latest research into food, health and disease prevention. In other words, it's topical as well as practical.

I hope, by the time you finish reading this book, you will have all the information and confidence you need to make sure you are eating the right combination of food to keep you fit, happy and well.

Chapter 1

The Essentials

Good nutrition is vitally important for our overall good health, but with so much conflicting advice in the media, and with so many different foods weighing down the supermarket shelves, how can we possibly be expected to choose which foods to eat and which to avoid?

In this chapter we'll go right back to basics and give you the facts to help you make sensible and realistic choices about what you eat.

If you want to know how to navigate your way through the food-labelling minefield, understand all those baffling buzz-words like 'antioxidants' or 'free-radicals', or you just want to have a firm grasp of the basics of nutrition, you'll find all the information you need in this chapter.

Not a week goes by without some new 'superfood' taking up column inches in the press, and the wealth of information now available to us can seem a little overwhelming at times. But it's not all bad. I have recently rediscovered the joys of the pomegranate, all because of the media attention it received about being a superfood. My granny used to love them, and it was a real treat to have one when I was a kid. But they were always so messy and difficult to eat, so *now I drink pomegranate juice – and it tastes gorgeous!*

Don't worry about getting bogged down in all the science and research behind the information in this chapter – the important thing is that we're here to arm you with all the facts you need to make good food choices for life.

✳ The food labelling battle

In 2008, the EU brought in compulsory food labelling to curb obesity. The new rules require all pre-packaged food to display amounts of sugar, salt, saturated fat, carbohydrates and calories on the front of packaging.

In the UK, there are two labelling systems in use at present:

1. The government-backed traffic light colour-coded labelling uses a red, amber or green symbol to signal whether foods contain high, medium or low levels of fat, saturated fat, sugar and salt.
2. The system of guideline daily amounts (GDAs), favoured by the food industry, gives the amount of calories, fat, saturated fat, sugar and salt in a serving, plus the percentage of the GDA.

What are guideline daily amounts (GDAs)?

GDAs appear on food labels as a guide to how much energy (calories) and the amount of key nutrients you should consume each day for a healthy diet.

They were developed by the UK's Institute of Grocery Distribution, a food and grocery industry research organisation. The GDAs for fat, saturated fat, sugar and salt are maximum target guidelines; the GDAs for carbohydrate and fibre are minimum target guidelines; and the GDA for protein is an average guideline. They are based on the needs of an average sedentary person – individual requirements will differ, depending on your weight, age, and the amount of exercise you do.

Energy

What exactly is energy?

You can't see energy but you can feel it – as heat. If you run up and down the stairs, then you feel a little warmer, don't you? That heat you've just made is the end result of a complex chain of biochemical reactions, which started with the food you ate. The protein, carbohydrate and fat in your food is broken down by enzymes in your gut into smaller molecules, absorbed, perhaps stored and then transported in your bloodstream to your body cells. Here the nutrients are converted into adenosine triphosphate (ATP): the energy 'currency' of your body. ATP consists of an adenosine 'backbone' with three phosphate groups attached. When one of these phosphate groups splits off, then energy is produced. Around one quarter of this energy fuels work (such as muscular movement); the rest is given off as heat. That's how your legs moved up and down the stairs. And that's why you also felt warmer.

Normally, you have enough ATP in your muscle cells to fuel a few seconds of exercise; after this your body breaks down glucose (from your blood or from stored glycogen in your muscles) and/or fat to make more ATP and therefore more energy.

$$ATP \longrightarrow ADP + P + ENERGY$$

Where do I get energy from?

Energy in food comes from carbohydrates, proteins and fats. Carbohydrates are the body's preferred fuel, although proteins and fats can also be converted into energy. Each nutrient provides different amounts of energy:

	1g provides:
Carbohydrate	4kcal (17kJ)
Fat	9kcal (38kJ)
Protein	4kcal (17kJ)
Alcohol	7kcal (29kJ)

You may be wondering if the source of the calories is important. If you are only considering weight loss or gain, the answer is no, it is the total *intake* of calories that is important. However, if you are talking about nutrition and health, it definitely does matter where your food calories come from. Generally, carbohydrates and proteins are healthier sources of calories than fats or alcohol.

What is a calorie?

A calorie is the unit used to describe the amount of energy in food. In scientific terms, it is defined as the amount of energy (heat) required to increase the temperature of one gram of water by one degree Celsius. A kilocalorie (kcal) is equal to 1,000 calories.

Calories, kilocalories, kilojoules – what's the difference?

All of these terms crop up on food labels, which can be a bit confusing! Suffice it to say that the scientifically defined calorie is a very small energy unit that is inconvenient to use because an average serving of any food typically provides thousands of these calories. For this reason, when speaking about food in the everyday sense, we say 'calorie' when we mean 'kilocalorie'. For example, a food label may declare a portion of the food contains 100 kilocalories, but we would probably say 100 calories.

You'll also see food energy measured in joules or kilojoules on food labels, which is the SI (International Unit System) unit for energy. One joule is the work required to exert a force of one newton for a distance of one metre. One kilocalorie is equivalent to 4.2 kilojoule.

How many calories do I need?

Your calorie needs depend on your genetic make-up, age, weight, body composition, daily activity and your lifestyle. They will differ from one day to the next and as you grow older. As a (very) rough guide, it's around 2,000 calories a day for women with a fairly inactive lifestyle and 2,500 for men.

To calculate more accurately the calories you need daily, you should take into account two main factors:

1. Your basal metabolic rate (BMR)
2. Your level of physical activity

Your BMR is the number of calories you burn at rest (to keep your heart beating, your lungs breathing, to maintain your body temperature, etc.). It accounts for 60 to 75 per cent of the calories you burn daily. Generally, men have a higher BMR than women.

The second factor, physical activity, includes all activities from doing the housework to walking and working out in the gym. The number of calories you burn in any activity depends on your weight, the type of activity and the duration of that activity.

Your daily calorie requirement is the sum of these two calculations – BMR plus energy used in activity.

Step 1: Estimate your basal metabolic rate (BMR)

(A) Quick method: As a rule of thumb, BMR uses 11 calories for every 1lb (½kg) of a woman's body weight and 12 calories per 1lb (½kg) of a man's body weight.

> **Women: BMR = weight in kg x 22 (alternatively, weight in pounds x 11)**
>
> **Men: BMR = weight in kg x 24 (alternatively, weight in pounds x 12)**
>
> **Example: BMR for a 60kg woman = 60 x 22 = 1,320kcal**

(B) Longer method: For a more accurate estimation of your BMR, use the following equations:

Age	Men	Women
10–18 years	(weight in kg x 17.5) + 651	(weight in kg x 12.2) + 746
18–30 years	(weight in kg x 15.3) + 679	(weight in kg x 14.7) + 479
31–60 years	(weight in kg x 11.6) + 879	(weight in kg x 8.7) + 829
60+ years	(weight in kg x 13.5) + 487	(weight in kg x 10.5) + 596

> **Example: BMR for a 60kg woman aged 31–60 years = (60 x 8.7) + 829 = 1,351kcal**

Step 2: Estimate your physical activity level (PAL)

Your physical activity level is the ratio of your overall daily energy expenditure to your BMR – a rough measure of your lifestyle activity.

- Mostly inactive or sedentary (mainly sitting): 1.2
- Fairly active (include walking and exercise once or twice a week): 1.3
- Moderately active (exercise two or three times a week): 1.4
- Active (exercise hard more than three times a week): 1.5
- Very active (exercise hard daily): 1.7

Step 3: Multiply your BMR by your PAL to work out your daily calorie needs

BMR x PAL
Example: daily energy needs for an active 60kg woman = 1351 x 1.5 = 2,027kcal

This figure gives you a rough idea of your daily calorie requirement to maintain your weight. If you eat fewer calories, you will lose weight; if you eat more then you will gain weight (see Chapter 2).

Do you need fewer calories as you get older?

As you get older, activity levels are often reduced, which causes a loss of muscle tissue, and so your energy requirements tend to decrease. But this isn't inevitable. Regular exercise (especially resistance training) can help reduce or prevent the 3.2kg decline in muscle mass generally observed with each decade of ageing.

Why do men need more calories than women?

Men generally have higher calorie requirements than women because they have more muscle tissue and, generally, weigh more. Muscle tissue has a big appetite for calories. The more muscle mass you have, the more calories you will burn. And the heavier you are (whether that's muscle or fat), the higher your metabolic rate.

Carbohydrate

Why do you need carbohydrate?

Carbohydrate is your main source of energy. Your brain, nervous system and heart need a constant supply of carbohydrate, in the form of blood glucose, in order to function properly. You also need carbohydrate to fuel your muscles. The carbohydrates in your food are stored as glycogen in your liver and your muscles. You can store up to 100g of glycogen (equivalent to 400 kilocalories) in the liver and up to 400g of glycogen (equivalent to 1,600 kilocalories) in your muscles. That's enough to fuel your energy needs for one day. The purpose of liver glycogen is to maintain steady blood-sugar levels. When blood glucose dips, glycogen in the liver breaks down to release glucose into the bloodstream. The purpose of muscle glycogen is to fuel physical activity. During exercise, glycogen in your muscles releases glucose, which is used for energy.

What is 'blood sugar'?

'Blood sugar' is the amount of glucose in your blood. It is expressed as milligrams per decilitre (1dl = 100ml) or millimoles per litre (mmol/l). Glucose is carried via the bloodstream to the body's cells, where it is used for energy. Blood-sugar concentration is kept within a very narrow range during rest as well as when you exercise: 70–110mg/dl or 3.9–6.1mmol/L. This allows normal body functions to continue. If your blood-sugar level drops below the normal range – 'low blood sugar' or hypoglycaemia – you may experience dizziness, faintness or even pass out, because the brain isn't getting enough glucose.

How much carbohydrate should I eat?

The government's panel of experts, the Committee on Medical Aspects of Food Policy, recommends a minimum 47–50 per cent of calories from carbohydrate. For an average woman eating 2,000 calories daily this works out at 230g of carbohydrate a day. For an average man eating 2,500 kcal, the guideline daily amount (GDA) is 300g. You will find these values on the GDA panel on food labels.

But the more active you are, the more calories and carbohydrate you need to fuel your muscles. In general regular exercisers need around five to seven grams of carbohydrate for each kilogram of their body weight. So a person weighing 60kg would need between 300 and 420g carbohydrate daily.

What's the difference between a simple and a complex carbohydrate?

Carbohydrates are traditionally classified as 'simple' and 'complex'. These terms refer to the size of the molecules, i.e. the number of sugar units they contain. Simple carbohydrates are very much smaller, comprising a single sugar (e.g. glucose) or two linked sugar units (e.g. sucrose). 'Complex' carbohydrates are bigger molecules, containing more than two linked sugar units, often thousands. They include starch (found in potatoes and cereals, for example) and fibre (found in fruit, vegetables and whole grains). But most foods contain a mixture of both types of carbohydrates, so it's impossible to classify foods as either 'simple' or 'complex'.

What's more, these terms tell you little about the effects

of that food on your blood-glucose level. It's a myth that complex carbohydrates provide 'slow-release' energy or simple carbohydrates provide 'fast-release' energy. In many cases, the precise opposite is true. For example, white bread (which contains complex carbohydrates) produces a rapid blood-sugar rise, while apples (containing simple carbohydrates) produce a gradual blood-sugar rise. Nowadays, carbohydrates are more commonly categorised according to their glycaemic index (GI).

What's the GI?

The GI is a ranking of foods from 0 to 100 based on their immediate effect on blood-sugar levels. It's a measure of how quickly the food is converted into blood glucose. The higher the GI, the bigger the blood-sugar rise. To make a fair comparison, all foods are compared with a reference food – normally glucose (GI 100) – and are tested in equivalent carbohydrate amounts. To measure the GI of a food, volunteers are given portions of food containing 50g carbohydrate and the rise in blood sugar is then measured over the next two hours, compared with glucose. Foods that produce a similar blood-sugar rise to glucose would get a high GI score; foods that produce a relatively small rise in blood sugar would get a low GI.

What do high GI and low GI mean?

Foods with a high GI (above 70) cause a rapid rise in blood-sugar levels. These include most refined starchy foods – potatoes, corn flakes, white bread and white rice – as well as sugary foods such as soft drinks, biscuits and sweets.

Foods with a low GI (below 55) produce a slower and smaller blood-sugar rise. These include beans, lentils, coarse-grain breads, muesli, fruit and dairy products.

And foods that contain no carbohydrate – meat, fish, chicken, eggs, oil, butter and margarine – have no GI value.

An easy GI guide

Low GI Foods	Moderate GI Foods	High GI Foods
Sweet corn	Pineapple	White bread and rolls, French bread and bagels
Sweet potato and yam	Raisins and sultanas	Regular sliced wholemeal bread
Most vegetables, e.g. cucumber, broccoli	Oatcakes and rye crispbread	Most breakfast cereals, e.g. corn flakes, crisped rice, bran flakes
Most fresh fruit, e.g. apples, pears, oranges, peaches, apricots, bananas, grapes, kiwi fruit, strawberries, mango	Whole-grain (brown) and basmati rice	Breakfast bars
Beans, chickpeas and lentils	Dried figs	Crackers and rice cakes
Low fat dairy products, e.g. milk and yoghurt; soya 'milk'	Chapatti	White rice
Pasta	Pitta bread	Gluten-free bread and pasta
Rye bread, coarse-grain bread, stone-ground wholemeal bread, breads containing oats/soy/cracked wheat/seeds	Rice noodles	Mashed, boiled and baked potatoes
Bulgur wheat, couscous, barley	Jam	Doughnuts
Fish, poultry and lean meat	Tinned fruit	Chips
Most fruit juice	Ice cream	Sugar
Nuts and seeds	Raisins	Soft drinks
Porridge, oatmeal, and muesli	Muesli bars	Sweets
Honey	Digestive biscuits	Most biscuits

Is a low GI diet healthier?

A 2008 study by Australian researchers, analysing the diets of nearly 2 million people around the world, found that a high GI diet increased the risk of diabetes, heart disease, stroke and various cancers. Studies at Harvard University in the US have correlated a low risk of diseases such as heart disease and diabetes with a low GI diet. In other words, people who eat lots of low GI foods such as whole grains, pulses, fruit and vegetables tend to be the healthiest. But that's not too surprising, as a low GI diet is in line with general healthy advice to eat more fibre, less saturated fat and sugar.

Staying on the move and taking plenty of exercise helps keep your body more sensitive to insulin. This means better blood-sugar control and fewer peaks and troughs. Studies at the University of Sydney in Australia have found that athletes produce much less insulin after eating high GI foods than non-active people.

What's the difference between the GI and glycaemic load (GL) diets?

Both GI and GL have been promoted as weight-loss diets. The difference between them comes down to portion sizes. The GI rules don't stipulate the amount of food eaten (eat low GI foods; avoid high GI foods), whereas the GL diet takes account of the portion size.

One big problem with the GI is that it can create a falsely bad impression of a food. For example, watermelon with its high GI (72) is off the menu on a low GI diet. But an average portion (120g), containing just 6g of carbohydrate, doesn't raise your blood-glucose level significantly. You would need to eat 8 slices (960g) to obtain 50g of carbohydrate – the amount used in the GI test.

Another drawback is that some high-fat foods (e.g. crisps, cake) have a low GI, which gives a falsely favourable impression of the food.

GL builds on the weaknesses of the GI diet. It is calculated by multiplying the GI of a food by the amount of carbohydrate per portion and dividing by 100.

GL = (GI x carbohydrate per portion) ÷ 100

So, a slice of watermelon has a high GI but a low GL:

GL = (72 x 6) ÷ 100 = 4.3

	GI value	GL value	Daily GL total
Low	0–55	0–10	0–80
Medium	56–70	11–19	80–120
High	71–100	> 20	> 120

✳ Why am I not losing weight on a low GI diet?

Several studies have found that low GI foods have no effect on people's hunger or overall calorie intake. A 2004 US study found that weight loss on a low GI diet was no different to that on a high GI diet. Clearly, a low GI value isn't a licence to eat freely; you still have to keep a rein on portion sizes. Low GI doesn't always mean filling or low-cal. Eat carb-dense foods (like cereals, bread, pasta) in moderation and fill up instead on fibre-rich foods with a high water content (fresh fruits, vegetables, salads).

Is sugar really bad for you?

Refined sugar provides a quick, simple source of energy but it doesn't contain other nutrients such as vitamins and minerals. Sugar is pure calories.

The biggest problem with sugar is that it damages teeth, especially kids' teeth. It feeds the bacteria in plaque and produces acids, which attack the enamel of the teeth and cause decay. Snacks, confectionery and fizzy drinks are the worst culprits because they are consumed between meals when the risk of damage to the teeth is highest. The more sticky a food, the more it will adhere to the teeth and the bigger the chances it has of causing decay. If you (or your kids) must have sugary foods or drinks, confine these to mealtimes when they'll do less damage.

Does sugar make you fat?

Many studies have linked sugar to obesity and related diseases. For example, a 2007 study from the Medical Research Council and the University of Cambridge found a strong link between the amount of sugar people ate and obesity. The main problem is that sugar raises the calorie density of foods and drinks. In other words, it adds to the amount of calories in food without adding bulk. It is often found with lots of saturated fat, for example in chocolates, cakes and biscuits, so it becomes easy to overindulge in foods and drinks with high sugar content.

✳ Sweet secrets

Sugar doesn't just come from obvious foods such as chocolate and cakes. Breakfast cereals, sauces, cereal bars and fruit bars contain lots of hidden sugar too. Check the label for words such as sucrose, glucose syrup, invert sugar and glucose – they're all forms of added sugar.

How much sugar can I eat?

Food experts recommend cutting down on the amount of sugar we eat. The Food Standards Agency (FSA) recommends adults should have no more than 60g added sugar a day – children should have even less (see table below). For food labelling, the GDA is 85g of *total* sugars, which includes natural sugars in fruit, fruit juice and milk, as well as added sugar.

When choosing sugar-rich foods, opt for those that provide you with energy but also with other nutrients. Go for fresh fruit, dried fruit, smoothies and fruit juice.

✳ How to cut down on sugar

○ Scrutinise labels. Opt mostly for foods containing less than 5–7g sugar per 100g (these may have green traffic light labels), and eat smaller portions of anything over 15g per 100 g (red traffic light labels).

○ Ditch the fizz – try swapping sugary and fizzy drinks for water.

○ Cut down on the amount of sugar in coffee and tea.

○ Swap snack bars that are high in sugar for fruit.

○ Opt for breakfast cereals with no or little sugar: Shreddies, Weetabix, porridge.

○ Rather than banning sweets and chocolate completely, limit them to certain clearly defined occasions. For example, allow one 'treat' on an agreed day of the week.

○ Keep any food and drink containing sugar mainly to mealtimes to reduce the risk of tooth decay.

○ Limit soft drinks, sweets, biscuits, cakes and puddings. Even artificially sweetened varieties encourage a liking for sugar.

○ Use more unprocessed foods that are

naturally sweet – like fresh and dried fruit –
they contain more vitamins and fibre.
- Give kids plain water to drink. If they're not
keen on it, try fruit juice diluted with water –
it's less sweet so will help re-educate their
palate for less sweet tastes generally.

How much sugar a day?

Age	Guideline Daily Amount (GDA)
4–6 years	40g (2½ tablespoons)
7–10 years	50g (3 tablespoons)
11–14 years	50g (3 tablespoons)
15–18 years	60g (4 tablespoons)
Adult	60g (4 tablespoons)

Are artificial sweeteners better than sugar?

Artificial sweeteners, such as aspartame, acesulphane K and
saccharin, have passed the scrutiny of food-safety commit-
tees worldwide. The UK government considers them safe
– although they're not allowed in baby foods – but some
scientists argue that high intakes may be linked with headaches, migraines and brain tumours. The current consensus
is that artificial sweeteners aren't linked with cancer.

There are other problems with artificial sweeteners. It is
thought that they might disrupt the body's natural ability to
'count' calories based on foods' sweetness, so limiting them
and having water instead of diet drinks is a good idea.

Also, they may not decay your teeth but they still encourage
intensely sweet tastes. Try to encourage a preference for more
natural sweetness from fresh or dried fruit, or just eat small
amounts of sweet foods, which have no artificial sweeteners.

Is it better to give kids fruit bars instead of confectionery?

Kids' fruit bars may sound healthier than confectionery because they claim to have no added sugar. But they're not! These bars are made from concentrated fruit purée and juice – in other words, sugar! These are no better for them than ordinary sugar and – due to their stickiness – just as damaging to their teeth.

Sugar content of various foods

Food	Amount of sugar
Chocolate bar	8 teaspoons
Can of cola	7 teaspoons
2 scoops ice cream	4½ teaspoons
1 pot of fruit yoghurt	3 teaspoons
Small bowl of Coco Pops	3 teaspoons
Small can of baked beans/ pasta shapes	2 teaspoons
2 biscuits	2 teaspoons
1 breakfast cereal bar	2 teaspoons
1 tablespoon tomato ketchup	1 teaspoon

✳ Check the label

To see if a product is high in sugar according to the Food Standards Agency recommendations, compare the amount per 100g with the following guidelines:

More than 10g is high
Less than 2g is low

How can I help my kids have healthy teeth?

○ Get them to brush their teeth with fluoride toothpaste twice a day, first thing in the morning and before bed.

○ Discourage sugary or sticky foods – sweets, chocolate, biscuits, raisins and other dried fruit and fruit bars – between meals. These leave residues on the teeth, increasing the risk of decay. Be aware that dried fruit is as potentially harmful to teeth as sweets!

○ If they must have sugary foods or drinks, it's better to have them in one go rather than sucking a packet of sweets or sipping a drink for an hour or more.

○ Encourage the drinking of acidic drinks with a straw. This reduces the contact of the drink with the teeth. Sugar-free drinks aren't necessarily better for children's teeth as they are quite acidic and can cause dental erosion.

○ Eating a small piece of cheese at the end of a meal or after a sugary or acidic snack helps counteract the harmful effects of sugar. Cheese is alkali and rich in calcium and neutralises the fruit acids.

Snacks and drinks that are safer for teeth

Snacks	Drinks
Fresh fruit	Water
Yoghurt	Milk
Cheese	Diluted fruit juice
Toast, plain or with Marmite, peanut butter or cheese	
Nuts	
Crudités with dips	
Savoury sandwiches	

FIBRE

What is fibre?

Fibre is a category of complex carbohydrates, found in plants, which cannot be digested by humans. There are hundreds of different fibres, which can be divided into two main kinds – insoluble and soluble. Most plant foods contain a mixture of the two. Insoluble fibre is the tough fibrous part of the plant. You'll find it in whole-grain foods, such as whole-wheat bread, whole-wheat breakfast cereals, whole-wheat pasta and whole-grain rice. Small amounts are also found in fruit and vegetables. Soluble fibre is found mostly in pulses (beans and lentils), oats, fruit and vegetables.

Is fibre good for you?

Both types of fibre have numerous health benefits. The insoluble kind is really important for helping your gut work properly, encouraging the natural rhythmical movements of the intestines and bowel, and speeding the passage of food to the bowel. Insoluble fibre reduces 'bad' LDL cholesterol levels and helps control blood-glucose levels by slowing glucose absorption. Low fibre intakes can lead to a sluggish gut, slow transit times (the time taken for food to pass through the gut) and often result in constipation. In the long term, a low-fibre diet can result in haemorrhoids, irritable bowel syndrome, polyps, diverticular disease and bowel cancer.

Can a high-fibre diet stop me getting cancer?

Possibly. In countries with traditionally high-fibre diets, diseases such as bowel cancer, diabetes and coronary heart disease are much less common than in the West. However, scientists are unclear as to whether these benefits are due to fibre itself or to other nutrients found naturally in fibre-rich foods. A 2003 study by Cancer Research UK and the Medical Research Council (the 'EPIC study') of more than half a million people in ten European countries found that people who ate the most fibre-rich food had the lowest incidence of bowel cancer while those with least fibre in their diets had the most cases of the disease. A 2007 study at the University of Leeds found that women eating 30g of fibre a day halved their risk of breast cancer compared with women on low-fibre diets (less than 20g). The US dietary guidelines recommend a minimum of three servings of whole-grain foods a day. One serving is one slice of wholemeal bread or a third of a cup of whole-wheat pasta.

Can fibre help me lose weight?

Yes. Fibre-rich foods are especially beneficial for weight control as they tend to fill you up and satisfy your appetite. They take longer to digest in your stomach, which means you feel full for quite a while after eating them. Fibre also expands in the gut, acting like a sponge, absorbing and holding on to water as it passes through you. A study of almost 3,000 adults in the US showed that over 10 years the people eating the most fibre gained less weight than those with the lowest intake of fibre. A 2007 study in Australia found that people who ate plenty of whole grains had a lower body mass index (see page 86), a smaller waist circumference and were less likely to be overweight.

Fibre also increases a food's 'chewing time' so that your body has time to register that you are no longer hungry. This will make you less likely to overeat and help you feel full for longer. Studies have shown that people who increased their fibre intake for four months ate fewer calories and lost an average of five pounds – with no dieting!

How much fibre should I eat?

The Food Standards Agency recommends an intake of 24g a day (this is the GDA you'll see on food labels). The average intake in the UK is around 16g a day, which is considerably less than the 80 to 130g eaten daily by our ancestors 5,000 years ago (according to estimates by scientists at the Paleobiotic Laboratory in New Orleans, US).

❋ How to eat more fibre

○ Include beans and lentils in your meals at least once a week, and then gradually increase to four times weekly or more. Use for making dahl, soups, salads, curries and pilafs. Add to Bolognese sauce, stews, chilli and shepherd's pie.

○ Aim for at least five portions of fruit and vegetables a day. Carry fresh fruit with you to have as a snack when you feel peckish.

○ Start the day with a bowl of porridge or breakfast cereals labelled whole grain, for example bran flakes, Shreddies, Shredded Wheat or Weetabix.

○ Swap white bread for whole-grain breads, such as wholemeal, rye and oatmeal.

○ Use whole grains in one-pot dishes, such as barley in vegetable stews and bulgur wheat in casseroles or stir-fries. Create a whole-grain pilaf with a mixture of barley, wild rice, brown rice, stock and herbs. Then add toasted nuts or chopped dried fruit.

I've heard of 'resistant starch' – is it the same as fibre?

Resistant starch is the part of starchy food (approximately 10 per cent) that resists normal digestion. It is found in beans, lentils, under-ripe bananas, pearl barley and bulgur wheat and is also produced when potatoes and rice have been cooked and then allowed to cool down. While not strictly speaking the same as fibre, it acts in a similar way. Bacteria in the large bowel ferment and change the resistant starch into short-chain fatty acids, which are important for keeping the cells lining the bowel healthy, and protecting them against cancer. These fatty acids are also absorbed into the bloodstream and help lower blood-cholesterol levels.

Protein

Why do I need protein?

Protein is needed for the growth, formation and repair of body cells. It forms part of the structure of every cell in your body, including muscle, skin, hair and nails. It is also needed for making enzymes, hormones and antibodies. Your body can't store protein, so it must be supplied on a daily basis from the foods you eat.

How much protein should I eat?

The amount of protein you need in your diet depends on your weight, age, lifestyle and activity. As a rough guide, the recommended intake for protein (measured in grams per kilogram of bodyweight) is 0.75g/kg/day. The guideline daily amount (GDA) is 45g for woman and 55g for men. The needs of children and adolescents also vary according to their age and weight (see page 73). Most people eat far more protein than they actually need, so deficiencies are rare.

Do athletes need extra protein?

Yes, athletes and regular exercisers have higher protein requirements than non-active people. Extra protein is needed to compensate for the increased muscle breakdown that occurs during and after intense exercise, as well as to build new muscle cells. Endurance athletes require between 1.2 and 1.4g protein per kilogram of body weight per day. That's 84 to 98g daily for a 70kg person. Strength athletes require 1.4 to 1.8g/kg, or 98 to 126g daily. However, protein supplements are not normally necessary – you can still get these levels of protein from a balanced diet.

What happens if I don't get enough protein?

If you don't eat enough protein for a few days or weeks, the body will simply adapt to a lower intake by 'recycling' existing proteins into new ones. However, if you were to continue eating a low-protein diet for several months, you might develop symptoms of protein deficiency: wasting and shrinkage of muscle tissue, oedema (build-up of fluids, particularly in the feet and ankles), anaemia and slow growth (in children). This condition is very rare in the West (even among vegetarians and vegans) but common in developing countries.

Is too much protein harmful?

Unlikely. As protein is found in so many foods, most people eat a little more protein than they need. This isn't harmful – the excess is broken down into urea (which is excreted) and fuel, which is either used for energy or stored as fat if your calorie intake exceeds your output.

Some athletes eat high-protein diets in the belief that extra protein leads to increased strength and muscle mass. But this isn't true – it is stimulation of muscle tissue through exercise, not extra protein, that leads to muscle growth. Again, the extra protein is unlikely to be harmful;

and contrary to popular belief, there's no evidence that high protein intakes damage the kidneys or liver in healthy people.

Can high protein diets help me lose weight?

Probably not. The main drawback of these diets is their very low level of carbohydrate. If the body doesn't receive enough carbohydrate, it will break down muscle tissue to make glucose. This causes muscle wastage, reduced metabolism and a build-up of ketones (by-products of protein metabolism). There is evidence to suggest that the heart may not function as well if its main source of fuel is ketones. A high intake of animal products (which is usually recommended in such diets) can also be high in saturated fats and cholesterol, which is associated with a range of conditions including heart disease. Recent research shows that weight loss over one year is not greater on a high-protein diet when compared with safer low-fat eating patterns.

Which are healthier – animal or vegetable proteins?

Animal protein sources (poultry, fish, meat, dairy products and eggs) generally provide a higher concentration of protein than vegetable sources (beans, lentils, nuts, grains, soya, Quorn). They also contain all eight essential amino acids (see page 29), whereas plant proteins may lack certain essential amino acids, making them less readily absorbed. However, this isn't necessarily a problem: eating a mixture of plant protein sources (such as beans on toast) enhances amino acid absorption.

Animal protein sources contain no fibre and some foods (meat and full-fat dairy products) may also contain high levels of saturated fat. Swapping some animal protein for vegetable protein is a good way to lower your saturated-fat intake and boost your intake of fibre. High intakes of animal protein increases acidity in the bloodstream, which is associated with increased bone mineral loss and osteoporosis risk. Substituting vegetable for animal protein will help cut your risk.

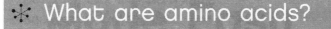

✳ What are amino acids?

Amino acids, the small components of protein, are often called the building blocks because they are used to repair muscle tissue. There are twenty different amino acids that, in different combinations, make up thousands of proteins.

A protein can consist of between fifty and tens of thousands of amino acids linked together. Eight amino acids must be provided by the diet (the 'essential amino acids'), while the body can make the others. But for your body to use food proteins properly, all eight essential amino acids have to be present. Animal proteins as well as soya and Quorn contain all eight essential amino acids. But plant proteins (pulses, cereals, nuts) contain smaller amounts, so these need to be combined together (e.g. beans on toast; lentils and rice; peanut butter on bread) to make a full complement of amino acids. The general rule of thumb is to have grains and pulses or nuts and grains together.

The protein content of various foods

Food	Protein (g)
Meat and Fish	
1 lean fillet steak (105g)	31
1 chicken breast fillet (125g)	30
2 slices turkey breast (40g)	10
1 salmon fillet (150g)	30
Tuna, canned in brine	24
Dairy products	
1 slice (40g) Cheddar cheese	10
2 tablespoons (112g) cottage cheese	15
1 glass (200ml) skimmed milk	7
1 glass (200ml) soya milk	7
1 carton yoghurt (150g)	6
1 egg (size 2)	8
Nuts and seeds	
1 handful (50g) peanuts	12
1 tablespoon (20g) peanut butter	5
Pulses	
1 small tin (205g) baked beans	10
3 tablespoons (120g) cooked lentils	9
3 tablespoons (120g) cooked red kidney beans	10
Soya and Quorn products	
1 tofu burger (60g)	5
1 Quorn burger (50g)	6
Grains and cereals	
2 slices wholemeal bread	6
1 serving (230 g) cooked pasta	7

Fat

Do I need any fat in my diet?

Although too much fat is harmful, some fat is essential – it makes up part of the structure of all your body cell membranes, your brain tissue, nerve sheaths and bone marrow, and cushions your organs. Fat in food also provides essential fatty acids (see below), the fat-soluble vitamins A, D and E, and is an important source of energy (calories), providing nine calories per gram.

How much fat should I eat?

The UK Department of Health recommends that fat provides no more than 33 per cent of your energy (calorie) intake, and saturated fat no more than 10 per cent of energy intake. This means the average woman should eat no more than 70g of fat a day, and no more than 20g of saturated fat – the amount supplied by a portion of oily fish, two tablespoons of olive oil, a pint of semi-skimmed milk and a handful of nuts. Men should have no more than 95g of fat and 30g of saturated fat daily. If you're trying to lose weight, reduce your fat intake by around 20g a day. Aim for most of your fat to be the 'good' unsaturated kind while avoiding 'bad' saturated and trans fats as far as possible.

✳ Easy ways to save on fat

1. Try using:

- Semi-skimmed or skimmed milk instead of full-fat milk.
- Chicken, fish and lean meat instead of processed meat, burgers, meat pies, pâté and sausages.

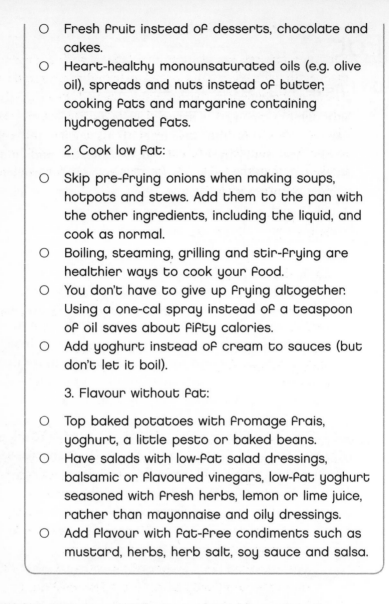

- Fresh fruit instead of desserts, chocolate and cakes.
- Heart-healthy monounsaturated oils (e.g. olive oil), spreads and nuts instead of butter, cooking fats and margarine containing hydrogenated fats.

2. Cook low fat:

- Skip pre-frying onions when making soups, hotpots and stews. Add them to the pan with the other ingredients, including the liquid, and cook as normal.
- Boiling, steaming, grilling and stir-frying are healthier ways to cook your food.
- You don't have to give up frying altogether. Using a one-cal spray instead of a teaspoon of oil saves about fifty calories.
- Add yoghurt instead of cream to sauces (but don't let it boil).

3. Flavour without fat:

- Top baked potatoes with fromage frais, yoghurt, a little pesto or baked beans.
- Have salads with low-fat salad dressings, balsamic or flavoured vinegars, low-fat yoghurt seasoned with fresh herbs, lemon or lime juice, rather than mayonnaise and oily dressings.
- Add flavour with fat-free condiments such as mustard, herbs, herb salt, soy sauce and salsa.

Bad fats, good fats – what are they?

Good fats are unsaturated – monounsaturates and polyunsaturates. They're found in nuts, seeds, olives (and their oils) and fish. Bad fats are saturated fat and trans fats. Eating less of them is vital, since too much can cause high levels of cholesterol, which contributes to heart disease.

Which are the bad fats?

Saturated fats are found in animal fats as well as products made with palm oil or palm kernel oil (a highly saturated fat). They have no beneficial role in keeping the body healthy – they raise blood-cholesterol levels and increase the risk of heart disease – so you do not actually need any in your diet. However, it would be impractical to cut out altogether, so stick to an intake less than the GDA: 30g for men and 20g for women.

Main sources include:

O   Fatty meats
O   Full-fat dairy products
O   Butter
O   Lard, shortening, dripping
O   Palm oil (appears as 'vegetable fat' on food labels)
O   Palm kernel oil (also appears as 'vegetable fat' on food labels)
O   Margarine, spreads, biscuits, cakes, desserts, etc. made with palm or palm kernel oil or 'vegetable fat'
O   Egg yolk

✳ Can saturated fats make you fat?

An Australian study found that polyunsaturated, monounsaturated and saturated fatty acids are broken down differently in the body and may not be used in the same way. Unsaturated fats (especially monounsaturated and omega-3 fatty acids from fish oils) may be more easily used up from fat stores during exercise than fats from other animal sources. This suggests that saturated fat may be more likely to go into and stay in fat cells than some forms of polyunsaturated fat and possibly monounsaturated fat.

What are trans fats?

Trans fats are even more harmful than *saturated fats*. Very small amounts occur naturally in meat and dairy products but most are formed artificially during the commercial process of hydrogenation, which converts unsaturated oils into solid spreads and shortenings (hydrogenated fats or oils). They can also form during deep-frying. These hard fats make pastries and biscuits crispy, cakes moist and fillings creamy, and increase the shelf life of fried foods.

What's 'bad' about trans fats?

Trans fats clog your arteries by increasing blood levels of LDL cholesterol ('bad' cholesterol) and lowering your HDL ('good') cholesterol. Intakes greater than 5g per day have been linked to a 30 per cent increased risk of heart disease, as well as having a harmful effect on the risk of diabetes, allergies and even certain cancers, possibly because the structure of trans fats is foreign when incorporated into body cells. A Harvard University study involving 32,826 nurses, published in 2007, found that those with the highest level of trans fats in their blood had triple the risk of heart disease compared with those with the lowest levels.

How much trans fat is it safe to eat?

There is no 'safe' level of trans fatty acids, according to the US Institute of Medicine, which recommends eliminating them completely. A trans fat ban has been put into effect in fast-food outlets in New York City and there are proposals to ban them from restaurants in California too. In the UK, the FSA recommends consuming no more than 4 to 5g per day. Unfortunately, figures for trans fats aren't given on labels, so minimise intake by avoiding foods with *hydrogenated oils* and *partially hydrogenated oils* on the ingredients list, in particular:

O   Margarine and spreads
O   Pastries, pies and tarts

- ○ Biscuits
- ○ Cereal bars, breakfast bars
- ○ Cakes and bakery products
- ○ Crackers
- ○ Ice cream, desserts and puddings
- ○ Fried food

✳ Some countries have banned trans fats – will the UK follow?

In 2006 the World Health Organisation recommended that governments around the world phase out hydrogenated oils. Greater consumer awareness of the health risks has resulted in many manufacturers in the UK, the rest of Europe and the US actively reformulating their products to replace and reduce the levels of trans fats. The FSA are encouraging manufacturers to reduce trans fat levels but have not brought in legislation banning the use of hydrogenated oils. In the US, food labels have had to list the trans fat content since January 2006. Denmark introduced trans fat legislation in 2003 by restricting the content of trans fats in all food products to a maximum of 2 per cent of the fat. In June 2007 Canada brought in similar trans fat limits and in July 2007 the Health Board of New York City imposed a ban on trans fats in the city's 40,000 restaurants. The EU is reluctant to adopt the policy across Europe but have conceded, in light of 'increased scientific evidence on the health hazards of trans fats that the intake of trans fats should be minimised'.

Good Fats	Bad Fats
Monounsaturated fats: olive oil, rapeseed oil, avocados, nuts, oil, peanut butter	Saturated fats: fatty meats, burgers, sausages, butter, palm biscuits, cakes, cheese
Polyunsaturated fats: sunflower oil, corn oil, sunflower margarine, nuts, seeds	Trans fats: some margarines and spreads, biscuits, pastries, pies, cakes, takeaway fried food
Omega-3 fats: sardines, salmon, mackerel, pilchards, walnuts, pumpkin seeds, omega-3 eggs	

What are good fats?

Monounsaturated fats help lower 'bad' LDL cholesterol levels (without affecting 'good' HDL), which cuts your heart disease and cancer risk. The Department of Health recommends an intake of up to 12 per cent of total calories.

They're found in:

O   Olive oil
O   Olive oil margarine
O   Rapeseed oil
O   Avocados
O   Soya oil
O   Peanuts, almonds, cashews
O   Peanut butter
O   Sunflower and sesame seeds
O   Mayonnaise

Polyunsaturated fats split into two groups – omega-3 and omega-6 – but the balance between them is often out of kilter in most people's diets. We eat ten times more omega-6s than omega-3s, while a ratio of 5:1 or less would be a healthier balance.

Omega-3 fatty acids fall into three main types: the short-chain fatty acid, alpha linolenic acid (ALA, found in plant sources) and the long-chain fatty acids, eicosapentanoic acid (EPA) and docosahexanoic acid (DHA), both found only in fish oils. DHA is needed in early life for the growing brain. EPA is needed for normal brain function and can reduce problems associated with ADHD, dyslexia and dyspraxia.

Omega-3s are a vital part of your diet:

○ **Omega-3s are part of every cell in your body.** The kind of fat you eat directly affects the fat present in the membrane of every cell in your body. Unless a certain amount of omega-3 is present in the cell membrane, it will not function as it should.

○ **Omega-3s are good for your brain.** EPA and DHA are a major part of brain membranes and are needed for the proper functioning of the brain. A New Zealand study showed that breast-fed babies (breast milk contains DHA and EPA) achieved higher scores in educational tests. UK studies have found low blood levels of EPA and DHA in children with dyslexia and ADHD.

○ **Omega-3s protect against heart disease and stroke.** EPA produces hormone-like substances called prostaglandins, which control the blood-clotting process. This can help prevent blood clots and reduce the risk of thrombosis. A 2007 study at Chicago University, US, found that omega-3s can help reduce blood pressure, thus lowering heart-disease risk. Omega-3s reduce the viscosity or stickiness of the blood. This means it can flow more easily through the smallest blood vessels. Omega-3s reduce blood-fats levels and help raise HDL cholesterol levels, which protect against heart attacks.

○ **Omega-3s keep you cheerful.** Omega-3s may stabilise mood and combat depression. US research has linked low intakes of omega-3s and low blood levels of omega-3s with depression.

○ **Omega-3s keep you young.** They may help prevent memory loss and prevent Alzheimer's disease.

- ○ **High omega-3 intakes may also reduce pain in people with rheumatoid arthritis.**
- ○ **Omega-3s boost exercise performance.** For regular exercisers, omega-3s increase the delivery of oxygen to muscles, and improve aerobic capacity and endurance. They also help speed recovery, reduce inflammation and joint stiffness.

You need only tiny amounts to keep you healthy but, as they are found in relatively few foods, many people struggle to meet the minimum requirement of 0.9g a day. Over the last fifty years dietary intake of omega-3s has declined by 50 per cent because we're eating less fish. And the meat we eat has a lower content of omega-3s these days due to changes in animal feeding. Aim to eat at least one portion (140g) of oily fish a week or one tablespoon of omega-3-rich oil daily.

The omega-3 content of various foods is shown in the table on page 40.

Main sources include:

- ○ Sardines, mackerel, salmon, fresh (not tinned) tuna, trout, herring
- ○ Walnuts and walnut oil
- ○ Pumpkin seeds and pumpkinseed oil
- ○ Flax seeds and flaxseed oil, rapeseed oil, soya oil
- ○ Sweet potatoes
- ○ Omega-3 enriched foods, e.g. eggs, bread, margarine and fruit juice

Should I give my child an omega-3 supplement?

The International Cod Liver Omega-3 Foundation suggests a daily intake of 200mg for children. An omega-3 supplement may benefit children with learning difficulties, including ADHD, dyslexia and dyspraxia. In particular, it may reduce problems associated with these conditions such as low attention, poor concentration, visual symptoms, mood swings, anxiety, sleep problems and eczema. However, there is no proof that supplements increase academic performance or IQ in other children. The best source of omega-3 fats for all children is from food: oily fish (sardines, mackerel, salmon, herring, pilchards, trout, fresh tuna), omega-3 eggs, walnuts and smaller amounts in other nuts, dark leafy green vegetables, sweet potatoes, pumpkin seeds and pumpkinseed oil, flaxseed oil, and omega-3 enriched foods (certain milks, margarine, bread and fruit juice).

What should I look for in an omega-3 supplement?

If you don't eat any food sources of omega-3s, then fish-oil supplements would be a realistic option. Choose a marine or fish oil, not a fish-liver oil (which contains high levels of vitamin A, harmful in excess), and a dose that provides around 500mg EPA and 100mg DHA daily. Have with food to reduce the fishy taste, although fruit-flavoured versions are available. Benefits are usually apparent after three months. You may then reduce the dose to half or one third.

Can Omega-3s make kids brainier?

Unlikely. While omega-3s are crucial for the development of the brain of an unborn child, there's no evidence that extra omega-3s after birth boost their IQ. That said, if you're planning on having a baby upping your intake now and during pregnancy will help provide the optimal conditions for the development of your child's IQ as well as their eyesight, hearing and mental health. Research has shown that omega-3 supplements may help children with specific behavioural and learning difficulties like ADHD, dyslexia or dyspraxia. A 2006 trial of 117 children aged 5 to 12 in a Durham primary school carried out by Oxford University researchers found that children with learning problems who took omega-3 supplements for three months improved their reading ability at more than three times the normal rate and more than twice the rate in spelling, over three months of treatment. There were also significant improvements in their ADHD symptoms.

Sources of omega-3 fatty acids

	g/100g	portion	g/portion
Salmon	2.5g	100g	2.5g
Mackerel	2.8g	160g	4.5g
Sardines (tinned)	2.0g	100g	2.0g
Trout	1.3g	230g	2.9g
Tuna (canned in oil, drained)	1.1g	100g	1.1g
Cod liver oil	24g	1 teaspoon (5ml)	1.2g
Flaxseed oil	57g	1 tablespoon (14g)	8.0g
Flax seeds (ground)	16g	1 tablespoon (24g)	3.8g
Rapeseed oil	9.6g	1 tablespoon (14g)	1.3g
Walnuts	7.5g	1 tablespoon (28g)	2.1g
Walnut oil	11.5	1 tablespoon (14g)	1.6g
Peanuts	0.4g	Handful (50g)	0.2g
Broccoli	0.1g	3 tablespoons (125g)	0.13g
Pumpkin seeds	8.5g	2 tablespoons (25g)	2.1g
Omega-3 eggs	0.2g	One egg	0.1g
Typical omega-3 supplement		8 capsules	0.5g

Omega-6 fatty acids include linoleic acid and gamma linolenic acid (GLA) found in vegetable oils such as sunflower and corn oil. These oils are widely used in food manufacturing. For this reason, it's relatively easy to eat plenty of omega-6s but most people aren't getting enough omega-3s.

This can result in an imbalance of prostaglandins ('mini' hormones' responsible for controlling blood clotting, inflammation and the immune system).

Main sources include:

○ Sunflower oil and sunflower oil margarine
○ Safflower oil, corn oil, groundnut oil, olive oil
○ Peanuts and peanut butter
○ Evening primrose oil
○ Sunflower and sesame seeds

Is cholesterol the same as fat?

Cholesterol is not fat. It is a waxy substance, which forms part of the membrane that surrounds every cell in your body. It is also used to make sex hormones such as testosterone and oestrogen. Most of the cholesterol in the body is made in the liver – and this is influenced by your genes, stress levels and the amount of saturated fat you eat. It is present in some foods such as eggs, offal and shellfish but, for most people, dietary cholesterol has very little effect on blood-cholesterol levels. What's important is the amount of saturated fat you eat. Once inside the body, the liver turns this fat into cholesterol.

What does a high blood-cholesterol level mean?

A high level of cholesterol in the bloodstream increases the risk of heart disease and artery disease. The amount of cholesterol in your blood is measured in units called millimoles per litre of blood, usually shortened to 'mmol/litre' or 'mmol/l'. A high blood-cholesterol level is judged to be above **5.0 mmol/l**, according to the National Institute for Health and Clinical Excellence (NICE). But knowing your cholesterol level isn't, on its own, enough to tell you your personal risk of heart disease. You also need to know your levels of lipoproteins. These are special molecules that transport cholesterol around the body. And it's the balance of these lipoproteins, rather than your overall total cholesterol level, that matters.

What does LDL and HDL cholesterol mean?

Around 70 per cent of the cholesterol in your blood is carried on *low-density lipoproteins* (LDL). These carry cholesterol from the liver to body cells, where the cells take as much cholesterol as they need, leaving any excess in the blood. If there's constantly too much LDL cholesterol left in the blood it can build up in the arteries, eventually causing blockages or breaking away to form clots – this is why it's often referred to as 'bad' cholesterol. A high level is defined by NICE as above **3.0 mmol/l.**

The remaining cholesterol in your blood is carried on *high-density lipoproteins* (HDL). This 'good' HDL picks up and removes excess cholesterol back to the liver for elimination from the body. High levels of HDL are associated with a low heart disease and stroke risk. The greatest danger is when someone has high levels of LDL cholesterol, and low levels of HDL cholesterol.

Usually, when you have your blood cholesterol measured, your GP will look at your total cholesterol level, plus your LDL and HDL cholesterol. Healthy levels of cholesterol are:

○ Total cholesterol – below 5 mmol/L
○ LDL cholesterol – below 3 mmol/L
○ HDL cholesterol – above 1 mmol/L

How can I lower my LDL cholesterol level?

Taking enough exercise, eating a healthy diet and not smoking will help lower your cholesterol levels. Cut down on saturated and trans fats. Replace with monounsaturated fats and omega-3 fats, both of which lower LDL levels. Eat more soluble fibre (found in oats, beans, lentils, fruit and vegetables), which stimulates the liver to produce more HDL, and more antioxidant-rich foods (see page 56), which help prevent

LDL being deposited on blood-vessel walls. See page 170 for more advice on nutrition and heart disease.

Vitamins and Minerals

Why do I need them?

Vitamins and minerals are substances that are needed in tiny amounts to enable your body to work properly and prevent illness. *Vitamins* support the immune system, help the brain function properly and help convert food into energy. They are important for healthy skin and hair, controlling growth and balancing hormones. Some vitamins – the B vitamins and vitamin C – must be provided by the diet each day, as they cannot be stored. *Minerals* are needed for structural and regulatory functions, including bone strength, haemoglobin manufacture, fluid balance and muscle contraction.

How much do I need?

The table on page 47 summarises the functions, best food sources, and requirements of twelve key vitamins and minerals.

What are RDAs?

The Recommended Daily Amounts (RDAs) listed on food and supplement labels are rough estimates of nutrient requirements, set by the EU and designed to cover the needs of the majority of a population. The amounts are designed to prevent deficiency symptoms, allow for a little storage, as well as covering differences in needs from one person to the next. They are not targets; rather they are guides to help you check that you are probably getting enough nutrients.

Should I take extra vitamins and minerals?

You don't have to. About 12 million people in the UK take vitamin and mineral supplements but, with the right food choices, you should be able to get all the vitamins and minerals you need to keep healthy and ward off disease. Indeed, there is solid evidence that diets rich in vitamins and minerals, and antioxidants in particular, lessen the risks of heart disease and cancer. But there's scant proof that vitamins in pills give the same benefits. A review by the US Preventive Services Task Force in 2003 concluded that while multivitamins are generally harmless and useful for filling the gaps in your diet, there's no scientific evidence that they will reduce your risk of chronic disease. No link either was found between supplements of individual vitamins or antioxidant combinations and cancer or heart disease. According to a 2002 Harvard University study, popping a pill can't erase the effects of a poor diet and a sedentary lifestyle. Foods contain additional important components such as fibre, phytonutrients and essential fatty acids.

How much is too much?

It's virtually impossible to overdose on vitamins and minerals from food. Problems of toxicity are more likely to arise from the use of supplements, so it is important to check the guidelines on the label and the safe upper levels (SULs) set by the FSA. The SUL is the amount that's unlikely to be harmful taken over a lifetime. The FSA warns against high doses of the following:

O   Vitamin A – high doses over prolonged time can cause liver damage, and birth defects in babies. Avoid supplements if you are pregnant or likely to become pregnant.

O   Vitamin B6 – taking more than 10mg a day on a long-term basis may lead to numbness and persistent pins and needles in your arms and legs.

O   Chromium in the form of chromium picolinate – may

cause cancer, although up to 10mg/day of other forms of chromium is unlikely to be harmful.

○ Vitamin C – although excess vitamin C is excreted in the urine, levels above 1000mg/day may result in stomach cramps, diarrhoea and nausea.

○ Iron – levels above 17mg/day may result in constipation and discomfort through an upset or bloated stomach.

○ Vitamin D – large doses can cause weakness, thirst, increased urination and, if taken for a long period, result in high blood pressure and kidney stones.

✳ What is the EU Food Supplements Directive?

The EU Food Supplements Directive, which came into effect in August 2005, is a piece of legislation that restricts the sale of certain vitamins and minerals. It determines what ingredients may be used and at what levels – only those forms of supplements that are included on an approved list can legally be sold in the UK and other EU countries. The aim is to ensure that all vitamin and mineral products on sale in the EU are approved by the European Food Safety Authority as safe, that they contain forms of vitamins and minerals that offer some benefit, and that they are clearly labelled.

I've read that some vitamin pills are bad for you – is this true?

A 2007 paper (which reviewed 68 different studies) published in the *Journal of the American Medical Association* hit the headlines in 2008 by suggesting that certain vitamin supplements (vitamins A and E and betacarotene) appear to increase death rates. The conclusion was misleading because the study combined the results of trials carried out on both healthy people and those already suffering from conditions such as heart disease. This makes the results very unreliable. Also, it is notoriously difficult for scientists to work out whether it's the vitamins or other factors (genes, lack of exercise, existing disease, smoking, drinking, etc.) that makes people die early. The bottom line is that while the benefits of taking vitamin supplements may be small, provided you stick to the recommended doses they are unlikely to do you harm either.

Can vitamin C stop you getting colds?

According to a 2007 review of 30 studies by Australian and Finnish researchers involving 11,350 people, taking vitamin C will not protect most people from the common cold. But taking extra vitamin C at the beginning of a cold may shorten its duration. They also found that people who are exposed to severe physical stress, such as marathon runners, may benefit.

Do anti-ageing supplements work?

No. Various supplements, such as idebenone, pycnogenol, Coenzyme Q10, acetyl l-carnitine and alpha lipoic acid claim to slow the ageing process. But there's no evidence they smooth out wrinkles or live up to their anti-ageing claims. The ingredients act as antioxidants (see page 53), mopping up age-promoting free radicals, but none have been successfully trialled on humans. Instead, spend your money on antioxidant-rich foods: fruit and veg (for vitamin C and betacarotene); nuts and vegetable oils (for vitamin E); and tea and red wine (for polyphenols).

Are vitamin injections better than pills?

There's no reason why vitamin injections should be any more beneficial than supplements and may even be dangerous. Injections of vitamins B6 and B12 claim to boost energy levels. But these benefits are unproven. Taking more than 10mg of B6 may lead to numbness and persistent pins and needles.

If I decide to take a supplement, what should I look for?

If you want to add multivitamins and minerals to your diet, look carefully at the label. Here are some guidelines to help you choose:

- It should contain around 23 key vitamins and minerals.
- The amounts of each vitamin should be between 100 and 1,000 per cent of the RDA stated on the label, but below the SUL.
- The amounts of each mineral should be no higher than the RDA because higher doses may be toxic.
- Choose multivitamins containing betacarotene rather than vitamin A – it is a more powerful antioxidant and, unlike vitamin A, is unlikely to have harmful side effects in high doses.
- Avoid supplements with unnecessary ingredients such as sweeteners, colours, artificial flavours and talc (a bulking agent).

Essential Guide to Vitamins and Minerals

Vitamin/ Mineral	How much?*	Why is it needed?	What happens if you get too little?	What are the best food sources?	Side effects of excessive intakes?
Vitamin A	700mcg (men) 600mcg (women) No SUL FSA recomm- ends	Needed for growth and develop- ment in children; helps vision in	Poor vision, dry skin, impaired growth in children, and an increased	Liver, cheese, oily fish, eggs, butter, margarine	Liver and bone damage; can harm unborn babies in pregnant women

	1,500mcg max	dim light; keeps the skin, hair and eyes healthy, keeps the linings of organs such as the lungs and digestive tract healthy, helping the body to fight infections	suscept-ibility to infection		(avoid during pregnancy)
Betacaro-tene	No official RNI SUL: 7mg	Converts into vitamin A, a powerful antioxidant that may protect against certain cancers and heart disease		Dark-green vegetables such as spinach and watercress, and yellow, orange and red fruits such as carrots, tomatoes, dried apricots, sweet potatoes and mangoes	Excessive doses of betacaro-tene can cause a harmless orange tinge to skin (revers-ible)
Thiamin	0.4mg/ 1,000 kcal 0.8mg for women; 1mg for men up to 50 years; 0.9mg for men over 50 years No SUL	Converts carbohyd-rates to energy; keeps nervous system and the heart healthy	Tiredness, a poor appetite, headaches, muscle fatigue, poor concentra-tion, dep-ression, irritability and heart	Whole-meal bread, fortified breakfast cereals, nuts, pulses, meat	Excess is excreted so toxicity is rare

	FSA recommends 100mg		problems		
Riboflavin	1.3mg (men) 1.1mg (women) No SUL FSA recommends 40mg	Converts carbohydrates, fats and protein into energy	Poor wound healing and skin, eye and mouth problems such as watery, bloodshot eyes, flaky and dry skin, chapped lips and a sore tongue	Milk and dairy products, meat, eggs	Excess is excreted (producing yellow urine!) so toxicity is rare
Niacin	13mg for women up to 50 years; 12mg for women over 50 years; 17mg for men up to 50 years; 16mg for men over 50 years SUL: 17mg	Converts carbohydrates, fats and protein into energy	Skin problems, weakness, fatigue and a loss of appetite	Meat and offal, nuts, milk and dairy products, eggs, wholegrain cereals	Excess is excreted; high doses may cause hot flushes
Pantothenic acid	There's no RNI; a safe intake for adults is considered to be 3–7mg	Releases the energy from food and keeps the nervous system and skin healthy	Deficiency very rare	Offal, fish, poultry, meat, whole grains, nuts, eggs, yoghurt, beans	Excess is excreted
Vitamin B6 (pyridoxine)	1.2mg for women; 1.4mg for	Metabolism of protein,	Deficiency rare	Liver, nuts, pulses,	Very high doses (over 2g/

	adult men SUL: 80mg	fat and carbohydrate; essential for the formation of red blood cells, antibodies and brain chemicals called neurotransmitters		eggs, bread, cereals, fish, bananas	day for months) may cause nerve damage, including numbness in the hands and feet
Folic acid	200mcg for women and men	Formation of red blood cells; works with vitamin B12 for growth and the reproduction of cells; good intakes when planning a pregnancy and in the first 12 weeks also protect against birth defects	Tiredness, and depression; low intakes prior to and during the early stages of pregnancy may increase the risk of having a baby with a neural tube defect such as spina bifida and cleft palate	Dark-green leafy vegetables, oranges, fortified breakfast cereals and bread, yeast extract, nuts and pulses	May mask symptoms of a B12 deficiency
Vitamin C	40mg SUL: 1000mg	Formation of collagen, which constitutes connective tissue; needed for healthy	Loss of appetite, muscle cramps, dry skin, bleeding gums, bruising,	Fruit and vegetables (e.g. raspberries, blackcurrants, kiwi, oranges,	Excess is excreted; doses over 2g may lead to diarrhoea and excess urine

		bones, blood vessels, gums and teeth; promotes immune function; helps iron absorption	nose bleeds, infections and poor wound healing. In severe cases scurvy develops	peppers, broccoli, cabbage, tomatoes)	formation; high doses (over 2g) may cause vitamin C to behave as a pro-oxidant (enhance free radical damage)
Vitamin D	No RNI for adults under 65 years; 10mcg for adults over 65. SUL: 25mcg	Needed for strong bones (with calcium and phosphorus), helps to absorb calcium, may help to prevent osteoporosis in later life	Reduced absorption of calcium (increasing the risk of osteoporosis deficiency in babies and toddlers, leads to soft bones and the development of rickets)	Sunlight; oily fish; eggs, liver, fortified breakfast cereals and margarine	Toxicity rare; very high doses may cause high blood pressure, irregular heart beat; excessive thirst
Vitamin E	No RNI in UK 10mg in EU SUL: 540mg	Antioxidant which helps protect against heart disease; promotes normal cell growth and development	Deficiency is rare	Vegetable oils; margarine, oily fish; nuts; seeds; egg yolk; avocado	Toxicity is rare
Calcium	1000mg (men) 700mg (women) SUL: 1,500mg	Builds bone and teeth; blood clotting; nerve and muscle	Increased risk of osteoporosis	Milk and dairy products; sardines; dark-green leafy	High intakes may interfere with absorption of other

		function		vegetables; pulses; nuts and seeds	minerals – take with magnesium and vitamin D
Iron	8.7mg (men) 14.8mg (women) SUL: 17mg	Formation of red blood cells; oxygen transport; prevents anaemia	Iron deficiency anaemia	Meat and offal; whole-grain cereals; fortified breakfast cereals; pulses; green leafy vegetables	Constip-ation, stomach discomfort; avoid unnecess-ary supple-mentation – may increase free radical damage
Zinc	9.5mg (men) 7.0mg (women) SUL: 25mg	Healthy immune system; wound healing; skin; cell growth	Loss of taste; frequent infections; poor wound healing	Eggs; whole-grain cereals; meat; milk and dairy products	Interferes with absorption of iron and copper
Magnesium	300mg (men) 270mg (women) SUL: 400mg	Healthy bones; muscle and nerve function; cell formation	Weakness; irregular heartbeat, muscle cramps	Cereals; fruit; vegetables; milk	May cause diarrhoea
Potassium	3500mg SUL: 3700mg	Fluid balance; muscle and nerve function	Muscle weakness; disorien-tation; irritability	Fruit; vegetables; cereals	Excess is excreted
Selenium	75mcg (men) 60mcg (women) SUL: 350mcg	Antioxid-ant which helps protect against heart disease and cancer	Reduced fertility; frequent infections	Nuts, cereals; vegetables; dairy products; meat; eggs	Nausea, vomiting, hair loss

Notes:

mg = milligrams (1,000mg = 1 gram)

mcg = micrograms (1,000mcg = 1mg)

*The amount needed is given as the Reference Nutrient Intake (RNI, Department of Health, 1991). This is the amount of a nutrient that should cover the needs of 97 per cent of the population. Athletes in hard training may need more.

SUL = Safe Upper Limit recommended by the Expert Group on Vitamins and Minerals, an independent advisory committee to the Food Standards Agency.

Antioxidants

What exactly are antioxidants?

Antioxidant nutrients include various vitamins (including betacarotene, vitamin C and vitamin E), minerals (such as selenium) and phytonutrients. They are found mostly in fruit and vegetables, seed oils, nuts, whole grains, beans and lentils.

Antioxidants help prevent or reduce cell damage caused by oxidation, a process that damages cells in the body and has been linked to the development of cancer, heart disease, Alzheimer's disease and Parkinson's disease.

✳ What are phytochemicals?

Phytochemicals are plant compounds that have particular health benefits. They include plant pigments (found in coloured fruit and vegetables) and plant hormones (found in grains, beans, lentils, soya products and herbs). Many phytochemicals work as antioxidants (see below), while others influence enzymes (such as those that block cancer agents). They may have the following benefits:

- ○ Fight cancer
- ○ Reduce inflammation
- ○ Combat free radicals
- ○ Lower cholesterol
- ○ Reduce heart disease risk
- ○ Boost immunity
- ○ Balance gut bacteria
- ○ Fight harmful bacteria and viruses

Are antioxidants good for me?

Yes, an antioxidant-rich diet is thought to protect against heart disease, cancer, premature ageing and other diseases. For instance, men who eat plenty of the antioxidant lycopene (found in tomatoes) may be less likely than other men to develop prostate cancer. Lutein, found in spinach and corn, has been linked to a lower incidence of eye lens degeneration and associated blindness in the elderly. Flavanoids, such as the tea catechins found in green tea, are believed to contribute to the low rates of heart disease in Japan.

✳ What are free radicals?

Free radicals are by-products of normal body processes, such as the conversion of food into energy. When oxygen is metabolised, it creates free radicals which steal electrons from other molecules, causing damage. The body can cope with some free radicals (and needs them to function effectively). However, an overload of free radicals can trigger the inflammation process that causes clogged arteries, thrombosis, heart disease and cancer. Oxidation can be accelerated by stress, cigarette smoking, alcohol, sunlight, pollution and other factors. Some of the conditions caused by free radicals include:

- O Acceleration of the ageing process
- O Increased risk of heart disease, as free radicals encourage low-density lipoprotein (LDL) cholesterol to stick to artery walls
- O Certain cancers, triggered by damaged cell DNA
- O Deterioration of the eye lens, which contributes to blindness
- O Inflammation of the joints (arthritis)
- O Damage to nerve cells in the brain, which contributes to conditions such as Parkinson's or Alzheimer's disease

Which foods contain the most antioxidants?

There are hundreds of different types of antioxidants and the best way to make sure you get enough of them is to eat at least five daily portions of fruits and vegetables. It's a good idea to eat as many different-coloured varieties every day. Good sources of antioxidants include:

- O **Allium sulphur compounds** – leeks, onions and garlic
- O **Anthocyanins** – eggplant, grapes and berries
- O **Betacarotene** – pumpkin, mangoes, apricots, carrots, spinach and parsley
- O **Catechins** – red wine and tea
- O **Copper** – seafood, lean meat, milk and nuts
- O **Cryptoxanthins** – red capsicum, pumpkin and mangoes
- O **Flavanoids** – tea, green tea, citrus fruits, red wine, onion and apples
- O **Indoles** – cruciferous vegetables such as broccoli, cabbage and cauliflower
- O **Isoflavanoids** – soybeans, tofu, lentils, peas and milk

- ○ **Lignans** – sesame seeds, bran, whole grains and vegetables
- ○ **Lutein** – leafy greens like spinach, and corn
- ○ **Lycopene** – tomatoes, pink grapefruit and watermelon
- ○ **Manganese** – seafood, lean meat, milk and nuts
- ○ **Polyphenols** – thyme and oregano
- ○ **Selenium** – seafood, offal, lean meat and whole grains
- ○ **Vitamin C** – oranges, blackcurrants, kiwi fruit, mangoes, broccoli, spinach, capsicum and strawberries
- ○ **Vitamin E** – vegetable oils (such as wheat-germ oil), avocados, nuts, seeds and whole grains
- ○ **Zinc** – seafood, lean meat, milk and nuts

Scientists at the USDA (United States Department of Agriculture) have compiled a database of 277 foods, ranked according to their ability to combat free radicals. Each food has an antioxidant 'score', called ORAC. It is short for Oxygen Radical Absorbance Capacity, and is a test-tube analysis that measures the total antioxidant power of foods and other chemical substances. If a food has a high ORAC score, then it means the food is high in antioxidants and is better at helping us fight diseases such as heart disease and cancer.

Top scoring sources of antioxidants

USDA data on foods with high levels of antioxidant phytochemicals

Food	Serving size	Antioxidant capacity per serving
Small red bean	½ cup dried beans	13,727
Wild blueberry	1 cup	13,427
Red kidney bean	½ cup dried beans	13,259

Pinto bean	½ cup	11,864
Blueberry	1 cup (cultivated berries)	9,019
Cranberry	1 cup (whole berries)	8,983
Artichoke hearts	1 cup, cooked	7,904
Blackberry	1 cup (cultivated berries)	7,701
Prune	½ cup	7,291
Raspberry	1 cup	6,058
Strawberry	1 cup	5,938
Red Delicious apple	1 apple	5,900
Granny Smith apple	1 apple	5,381
Pecan	1oz	5,095
Sweet cherry	1 cup	4,873
Black plum	1 plum	4,844
Russet potato	1, cooked	4,649
Black bean	½ cup dried beans	4,181
Plum	1 plum	4,118
Gala apple	1 apple	3,903

Source: Oxygen Radical Absorbance Capacity of Selected Foods –
2007; Nutrient Data Laboratory, Agricultural Research Service,
United States Department of Agriculture, November 2007.

Should I take antioxidant supplements?

Research is divided over whether or not antioxidant supplements offer the same health benefits as antioxidants in
foods. Evidence suggests that antioxidant supplements
don't work as well as the naturally occurring antioxidants
in foods such as fruits and vegetables. For example, vitamin
A (betacarotene) has been associated with a reduced risk
of certain cancers but an increase in others, such as lung
cancer in smokers. A study examining the effects of vitamin

E found that it didn't offer the same benefits when taken as a supplement. Also, antioxidant minerals or vitamins can act as pro-oxidants or damaging 'oxidants' if they are consumed at levels significantly above the recommended amounts for dietary intake.

A well-balanced diet, which includes antioxidants from whole foods, is best. Your diet should include five daily portions of fruit and vegetables. If you decide to take supplements, choose one that contains all nutrients at the recommended levels.

Why does the government recommend 5 a day?

Research around the world indicates that people who consume at least five portions (400g) of fruit and vegetables in their diet have the lowest risks of degenerative diseases, such as cancer, diabetes, heart disease, and stroke and bowel disease. They are also less likely to be obese, have lower levels of cholesterol and lower blood pressure. The Department of Health guidelines recommend that adults eat at least five portions of fruit and vegetables every day. But the 2005 Health Survey for England found that only 26 per cent of men and 30 per cent of women were meeting this target – the average intake was just less than three portions a day.

Some other countries recommend higher intakes: in Australia the authorities recommend five portions of vegetables and two portions of fruit every day; US authorities recommend two portions of fruit and two to three (large – 120g) portions of vegetables from five different categories.

What counts towards your 5 a day?

All fruit and vegetables, including fresh, frozen, canned, dried and pure juices, count. The only exception is potatoes, which are a starchy food and so aren't included in the recommended 5 a day. Meanwhile, no matter how much you drink, a glass of pure juice only counts as one portion because it's not a good source of fibre and the juicing process squeezes out all the natural sugars that are normally found between the cells of the fruit or veg, with the result they're less healthy for teeth.

What's a portion?

On average, a portion of fruit or veg is equivalent to 80g. Here are some examples of what counts as one portion:

- 1 apple, banana, pear, orange or other similar-sized fruit
- 2 plums, satsumas, kiwi fruit or other similar-sized fruit
- Half a grapefruit or avocado
- 1 large slice of melon or fresh pineapple
- 3 heaped tablespoons of vegetables, beans or pulses
- 3 heaped tablespoons of fruit salad or stewed fruit
- 1 heaped tablespoon of raisins or sultanas
- 3 dried apricots
- 1 cupful of grapes, cherries or berries
- 1 dessert bowl of salad
- 1 small glass (150ml) of pure fruit juice

Are organic fruit and vegetables really better for you?

Until recently, there wasn't much evidence that organic food is healthier than non-organic; most people bought it because they liked the idea of sustainable agriculture, produce grown without chemicals and animals free of antibiotics. But now scientists are finding proof that organic food is, in fact, more nutritious. One of the best comes from a ten-year study published in 2007, which found that organic tomatoes had almost twice the amount of antioxidant nutrients compared with non-organic tomatoes. According to the research carried out at the University of California, levels of flavanoids, quercetin and kampferol were 79 and 97 per cent higher respectively. There have been other studies too. In 2007 a

European Union research programme reached similar conclusions about organic peaches, apples and tomatoes. They all contained higher levels of vitamin C and flavanoids. Another 2007 US study found that organic kiwis had significantly higher levels of vitamin C and polyphenols.

How can you make kids eat more fruit and vegetables?

Getting children to eat their 5 a day can be a struggle. But it's worth it as these foods are rich in vitamins and minerals, which help keep them healthy and boost their immunity. Five a day will help protect against colds, infections, constipation and degenerative conditions such as heart disease, stroke and certain cancers as they get older. Here's how to do it.

Set a good example yourself: Children are more likely to eat fruit and vegetables if they see you enjoying these foods daily and if there's a plentiful supply in the house.

Start a chart: Use a star reward chart to meet their 5-a-day target, giving one star for each daily portion of fruit and veg.

Get them in the kitchen: Let your children help wash, peel and cut vegetables. When they feel involved with meal planning and preparation, they are more likely to try new vegetables.

Take them shopping: Get children involved with the shopping – let them choose a new variety of fruit or vegetable (and then, hopefully, eat it!).

Don't force it: Won't eat spinach or sprouts? Don't fret if your children won't eat a wide range of vegetables. They can get the key nutrients – vitamin C and betacarotene – from strawberries and carrots. As their tastes develop, they will start to like other vegetables.

Add vegetables to pizzas: Let children decorate their own pizzas with a selection of peppers, sweet corn, courgettes, mushrooms, tomatoes and pineapple. Or mix finely chopped or puréed vegetables into the tomato sauce before topping the pizza base.

Hide 'em: You can get children to try a new vegetable if you mix it with a food they already like, such as mashed potato (try adding swede, parsnip, cabbage or spinach), soup, curry or macaroni cheese.

Eat 'em raw: Carrot and cucumber sticks, pepper strips, baby sweet corn and cherry tomatoes make lunchbox foods or teatime nibbles. Serve with hummus, salsa or a cheesy dip. Younger children who refuse most vegetables will often eat 'finger' vegetables.

Make snacks healthy: Establish healthy snack habits, making fresh fruit the norm for at least one snack daily. Apple slices, grapes and peeled satsumas are all good choices.

Start early: Get them to have one fruit portion at breakfast. Top breakfast cereal with sliced bananas, grated apple or a handful of raisins.

Eat dessert first: If your children are too hungry to wait for supper, give them dessert first – apple slices, grapes, melon – to stave off their hunger pangs and reach their daily 5-a-day target.

Display fruit: If fruit is on display – say in a fruit bowl – in a place your children can easily reach, they're more likely to grab them as they go past.

Mix with yoghurt: Mix berries or chopped soft fruit such as bananas with plain or fruit yoghurt. Alternatively, layer chopped or mashed fruit with yoghurt in tall sundae glasses.

Fruit cut into bite-sized pieces will be more attractive than whole fruit for younger children. Make a platter of bite-sized pieces of fruit and let your children dig in.

If your child must snack in front of the television, give them a bowl of grapes, cherries or sliced apples. Without realising it, they could get a couple of their 5 a day while watching their favourite programme.

Salt

We're told to cut down on salt – why?

Too much salt can cause raised blood pressure, which triples the risk of heart disease and stroke. Excess salt also leaches calcium from the bones, making them weaker; it aggravates asthma, puts stress on the kidneys and increases the risk of stomach cancer. Populations with a high average salt intake have a higher average blood pressure and higher levels of hypertension (high blood pressure).

Most people consume much more salt than they need – around six times more to be exact! The government estimates that cutting salt intake by a third would lead to a 10 per cent drop in heart disease cases and save around 35,000 lives each year.

Should I cut out salt completely?

No, because a small amount of salt in your diet is crucial for health. It helps regulate the volume of blood circulating in the body and the movement of fluid between cells as well as helping cells to take in nutrients from the blood and helps muscles contract. In all, you need 575mg sodium (1.4g salt) daily.

How much salt should I have, then?

The government's Committee on Medical Aspects of Food Policy recommend a maximum intake of 4g of salt a day (or 1,600mg of sodium) in order to prevent chronic disease. But the Food Standards Agency (FSA) recognises it may be difficult for many people to reduce their salt intake to the ideal level, given our current food supply, and advises reducing salt intake to less than 6g of salt a day (approximately 2,300mg of sodium a day) as a first step towards reaching the recommended levels. This is approximately 1½ teaspoons of salt. Children under seven should have no more than 3g of salt a day. Those between seven and ten should have no more than 5g daily and those aged eleven-plus no more than 6g daily.

Has the FSA's salt campaign worked?

There are promising signs that the average salt intake is starting to fall since the start of the national salt campaign. Between 2001 and 2008 the average fell from 9.5g to 8.6g. This is most likely because many food manufacturers have reduced the amount of salt they add to processed foods, in particular bacon, ham, sausages, burgers, crisps, baked beans, bread, pizza, cakes, butter and cereals. The FSA has set voluntary salt targets for these foods.

What's the easiest way to cut down on salt?

As a rule of thumb, try to avoid foods containing more than 1.25g salt per 100g. Three-quarters of the salt we eat comes from processed food, such as meat products (ham, bacon, sausages and burgers), bread, soups, sauces, cheese, ready-meals, pizzas, baked beans, breakfast cereals and biscuits.

O   Avoid adding salt to cooking and at the table.

O   Buy 'low salt' or 'salt free' versions of commonly used foods.

O   Use herbs and spices such as garlic, oregano and lemon juice to add flavour to meals.

O   Choose reduced-salt versions of tinned foods, such as pasta shapes in tomato sauce and baked beans.

O   Eat less burgers, sausages and chicken nuggets.

O   Swap salty snacks like crisps for unsalted nuts, plain popcorn, dried fruit, grapes and satsumas.

O   Cut back on ready-meals, takeaways and ready-made sauces.

O   Check labels on food to check how much salt is listed on the packaging. Try to choose foods containing less than 0.25 g salt per 100g.

Salt contents of various foods (per typical portion)

Chicken nuggets	1.8g
Pizza	1.3g
Can of baked beans	2.5g
Doughnut	1.2g
Hamburger	2.0g
Milk shake	0.5g
Frosties cereal	1.5g
Tinned spaghetti	2.3g
2 fish fingers	1.3g
Pasta sauce	1.0g
Crisps	0.6g
Shepherd's pie ready-meal	1.9g

The Guideline Daily Amount for salt for children and adults

Age	GDA
4–6 years	3g
7–10 years	5g
11+ years	6g
Adults	6g

Should children also cut down on salt?

Like adults, children should also avoid eating too much salt. This is because salt can raise blood pressure in children as well as in adults. And children are particularly vulnerable to the effects of salt. A 2006 study at St George's Medical School, London, found that reducing children's salt intake significantly reduces children's blood pressure.

So it's important to keep an eye on how much salt your child is consuming. Children under seven should have no more than 3g of salt a day. Those between seven and ten should have no more than 5g daily and those aged eleven-plus no more than 6g daily.

✳ Check the label

To see if a product is high in salt, according to the Food Standards Agency recommendations, compare the amount per 100g with the following guidelines (or check the traffic light label found on certain products):

Salt: More than 1.25g is high
          Less than 0.25g is low
Sodium: More than 0.5g is high
          Less than 0.1g is low
One gram of sodium is equivalent to 2.5g of salt.

Water

Why do I need to drink water?

Fluid cushions your nervous system, acts as a lubricant for your joints, keeps your eyes and mouth moist, helps you swallow, allows you to absorb nutrients, and helps get rid of waste. On top of that it helps regulate your temperature – you sweat when you get too hot. You need to top up your fluid levels frequently because you lose water through sweat, breathing and urine. Dehydration can make you feel tired and lethargic, and will decrease your capacity for exercise.

Do I really need eight glasses of water a day?

While there's no doubt that maintaining your fluid levels is very important, the belief that we need eight glasses of water a day to stay healthy is a myth. A major review of studies from the University of Pennsylvania in the US, which hit the headlines in 2008, concluded that there is no clear evidence of any benefits from drinking so much. Most people can rely on their sense of thirst as a good indicator of when they should drink. The exception to this is the elderly and people who exercise a lot, who should drink regularly even if not feeling thirsty. Though 1.5 to 2 litres of water is the oft-quoted amount needed to keep you hydrated, you shouldn't be too concerned about sticking to it rigidly. From a hydration point of view, it does not matter where you get your liquid from – coffee, tea, fruit juice, soup, squash and milk all count towards the total.

Can drinking extra water help flush out toxins?

There is no solid evidence that drinking plenty of pure water is good for the skin, wards off weight gain or helps rid the body of toxins. Healthy kidneys are particularly efficient at removing toxins. Drinking more water than you actually need won't remove any more toxins, it will just mean more trips to the loo!

Do coffee and tea really count?

The latest research on health and hydration indicates that even tea and coffee count towards your fluid intake. While it's true that the caffeine in tea and coffee has a mild diuretic (urine increasing) effect, there is a net gain of fluid when you drink a cup. The diuretic effects of caffeine are greatly outweighed by the fluid you get – you don't need to drink extra water to compensate.

Is mineral water better for me than tap water?

Mineral water contains small amounts of minerals, but not enough to make a significant contribution to your diet. Tap water is no less 'pure' and no worse for you than bottled mineral water. In fact, a Thames Water survey revealed that two-thirds of Britons prefer tap water to bottled water. And a 2008 *Which?* survey concluded that bottled water is 'expensive and bad for the environment'. Half the people surveyed could not tell the difference between tap and bottled water. UK tap water contains safe levels of chlorine to make sure it's clean. But placing a covered jug of water in the fridge for a few hours before drinking can reduce the chlorine taste.

How can you tell whether you're drinking enough liquids?

The colour of your urine is probably the easiest way to monitor whether you're getting enough liquids. It should be clear and copious. If you find your urine is dark in colour and you're only passing small volumes, you need to drink more.

Is it possible to drink too much water?

Drinking a lot of water (and that means more than 4 to 6 litres) over a short time can upset the body's sodium balance, and cause a potentially fatal condition called hyponatraemia, or water intoxication. This sometimes happens in long-distance runners because they often consume a lot of water and lose a lot of salt through sweat. Also, exercise releases an anti-diuretic hormone, so urine output is reduced, limiting the body's ability to correct the imbalance. As the water content of the blood increases, the salt content is diluted. Consequently the amount of salt available to body tissues decreases, which can lead to problems with brain, heart and muscle function. Initial symptoms of over-hydration include dizziness, nausea, bloating, lapses in consciousness and seizures due to swelling of the brain. However, these symptoms are also associated with dehydration – so it's important to be aware of how much you are drinking. If you plan to exercise for more than four hours in warm weather drink no more than 800ml per hour, be guided by thirst (instead of forcing yourself to drink) and sip a sports drink containing sugar and salt instead of plain water.

What are the healthiest drinks to give children?

The safest drinks for children's teeth are water and milk. Flavoured milk and milkshakes with less than 5 per cent added sugar will not harm teeth either.

Fruit juice is a healthy drink – it contains valuable vitamins and minerals and can count as one portion a day towards the five-a-day target – but its high acidity may cause acid erosion, resulting in a thinning of the tooth enamel. Try to keep fruit juice to mealtimes, when the sugars and acids in the drink are less harmful.

Smoothies contain the whole fruit so they are a good way of boosting vitamin, mineral and fibre intakes, and count as one of a child's five fruit and veg portions a day. Check the label to make sure it contains no added sugar or additives.

Avoid giving children squash, juice drinks and fizzy drinks as these contain high levels of added sugar and acid, which are both bad for teeth. Also, if children drink them regularly, sugary drinks add unwanted calories and encourage obesity.

Alcohol

I'm confused about alcohol – is it beneficial or harmful?

This depends mainly on how much you drink. Alcohol in moderation (up to two units a day) is associated with a lowered heart disease risk, due in part to its ability to increase levels of 'good' HDL cholesterol and reduce platelet stickiness. Red wine is thought to be particularly good for you because it contains polyphenols, saponins and a compound called resveratrol, all of which help lower 'bad' cholesterol and stop blood platelets from clumping together, thus affording greater heart disease protection. Pinot Noir grapes have especially high levels of resveratrol, and grapes grown in the Chilean valleys, Bordeaux and Burgundy in France have the best levels of their nutrient. Other super-nutrients in wine also have antioxidant effects, helping increase levels of 'good' HDL cholesterol and lowering blood pressure. But these benefits seem to be limited to men over forty and women over fifty. They do not apply to younger people – alcohol may severely impair their physical and mental development.

But isn't alcohol a toxin?

Yes, alcohol is a toxin and affects every body cell and every system in the body. It is a depressant drug and affects your co-ordination, self-control, judgement and reaction times. The risk of raised blood pressure, cirrhosis, certain cancers (including breast cancer), stroke, brain damage and other diseases becomes greater with increased alcohol consumption. 'Binge drinking' (drinking heavily over a short period of time or drinking continuously over a number of days or weeks) can be especially harmful. It can result in confusion, blurred vision, poor muscle control, nausea, vomiting, sleep, coma or even death.

How much alcohol is it safe to drink?

The UK Department of Health advises a maximum of three units a day and fourteen units a week for women; and a maximum of four units daily and twenty-one units weekly for men. Drinking more than these levels increases your health risk.

What's a unit?

A single unit contains 10g of alcohol, equivalent to 125ml (4fl.oz) of a wine that is 8 per cent alcohol by volume (ABV). But this measure was devised in the 1980s when many popular wines were only around 8 per cent alcohol. Nowadays most wines are at least 12 per cent alcohol and the size of a drink served in some bars and restaurants or even at home may be much bigger than a 'standard' measure.

✳ Units for alcoholic drinks

Drink	Volume	Strength	Units
Normal beer/lager/cider			
half a pint	284ml	4%	1
large can/bottle	440ml	4.5%	2
Strong beer/lager/cider			
half a pint	284ml	6.5%	2

large can/bottle	440ml	6.5%	3
Wine			
small glass	125ml	12.5%	1.5
medium glass	175ml	12.5%	2
large glass	250ml	12.5%	3
bottle	750ml	12.5%	9
Spirits			
single shot	25ml	40%	1
bottle	750ml	40%	30
Alcopops			
bottle	275ml	5%	1.5

Source: Office for National Statistics

What causes a hangover?

The symptoms of a hangover are due mainly to acetaldehyde, the by-product of alcohol breakdown. It's a poison, which the body eventually turns into acetic acid (vinegar) and then into water and carbon dioxide. But if you consume alcohol faster than your body breaks it down, levels of acetaldehyde rise and you feel ill. Alcohol also causes dehydration. This is why several glasses of water before going to sleep will lower the chances of next-day misery. A third cause of hangovers is the presence of 'congeners' in the alcoholic drink. These include colours and other additives. Generally speaking, the darker the drink, the more likely it is to produce a hangover: red wines, port and brandy tend to be the biggest culprits.

✳ Sensible drinking guidelines

Drink spacers – intersperse alcoholic drinks with water, diluted juice or other non-alcoholic drinks. Extend your alcoholic drink with water, low-calorie mixers or soda water.

Keep a tally – it's easy to drink more than you should without realising it. Set yourself a safe limit, avoid top-ups, and count the units in each drink.

Make excuses – do not feel obliged to drink excessively, even if your friends press you: tell them you are training the next day or that you are driving.

Eat – do not drink on an empty stomach as this speeds alcohol absorption. Try to eat something first or reserve drinking for mealtimes. Food slows down the absorption of alcohol.

Put down your glass – if you hold your drink in your hand at a party, you will drink more quickly than if you put it down on a table. At mealtimes, keep the wine bottle out of reach/sight – it will be less tempting to keep refilling your glass.

Why does alcohol affect me more at lunchtime?

Having a drink at lunchtime has more effect than during the evening because you make fewer alcohol-breaking enzymes during the day. So one drink can act like two. Pre-menstrual hormone changes have a similar effect.

Healthy eating for children

How can I persuade my children to eat healthily?

Children are more likely to do as you do. If children see their parents enjoying eating healthy foods and taking regular exercise, they are likely to do the same. A 2004 study carried out by University College London found that the more often parents ate fruit and vegetables, the more likely it was their children would have a high intake.

Being a good role model is the best way to encourage good habits in your children. What children see at home makes a big impact on their lifelong eating and exercise habits. If you opt for ready-meals and takeaways, you can't expect your children to relish regular helpings of fruit and vegetables.

Here are some ways of getting children to eat a healthier diet:

○ Explain the benefits of eating more healthily. This should be in terms that your children can understand and directly relate to, e.g. having more energy to play football; feeling more refreshed in the morning.

○ Put children in control of some of their food choices, e.g. allow them to choose which vegetables to eat; let them suggest a new meal.

○ Make some realistic goals, e.g. to eat two pieces of fruit a day; to try a new vegetable; to replace crisps with an apple or a handful of nuts.

○ Set up a reward system, e.g. award a star or sticker for each healthy eating behaviour. When, say, ten stars have been earned, choose a reward (preferably non-food, such as a new toy or a special trip) that has been agreed upon in advance.

- Increase the range of foods in your family's repertoire — try new recipes and offer healthy snacks.
- Set a good example yourself — don't show reservation in trying new foods.
- Praise children for trying a new food. Even if they don't like it, encourage them to explain why. Try the motto: 'taste before you judge' – it always works with my children who end up eating the lot!
- If a new food or dish is rejected initially, leave it for a while then reintroduce it a week or so later. Children will eventually like healthy foods if they are continually exposed to them.

What should kids be eating?

Approximate daily nutritional needs of children

Food Group	Number of portions each day	Food	Portion size (5–8 years)	Portion size (9–12 years)
Vegetables	3		The amount a child can hold in their hand	
		Broccoli, cauliflower	1 or 2 spears/florets	2 or 3 spears/florets
		Carrots	1 small carrot	1 carrot
		Peas	2 tablespoons	3 tablespoons
		Other vegetables	2 tablespoons	3 tablespoons
		Tomatoes	3 cherry tomatoes	5 cherry tomatoes
Fruit	2		The amount a child can hold in their hand	
		Apple, pear, peach, banana	1 small fruit	1 medium fruit
		Plum, kiwi fruit,	1 fruit	1 or 2 fruits

		satsuma		
		Strawberries	6	8–10
		Grapes	8–12	12–16
		Tinned fruit	2 tablespoons	3 tablespoons
		Fruit juice	1 small glass	1 medium glass
Grains and potatoes	4–6		The size of a child's fist	
		Bread	1 small slice	1 slice
		Rolls/muffins	½ a roll	1 roll
		Pasta or rice	3 tablespoons	4 tablespoons
		Breakfast cereal	3 tablespoons	4 tablespoons
		Potatoes, sweet potatoes, yams	1 fist-sized	1 fist-sized
Calcium-rich foods	2	Milk (dairy or calcium-fortified soya milk)	1 small cup	1 medium cup
		Cheese	Size of 4 dice	Size of 4 dice
		Tofu	Size of 4 dice	Size of 4 dice
		Tinned sardines	1 tablespoon	1–2 tablespoons
		Yoghurt/fromage frais	1 pot	1 pot
Protein-rich foods	2		Size of a child's palm	
		Lean meat	1 slice (40g)	1–2 slices (40–80g)
		Poultry	2 thin slices/1 small breast	2 medium slices/1 breast
		Fish	Half a fillet	1 fillet
		Egg	1	1 or 2
		Lentils/beans	2 tablespoons	3 tablespoons

		Tofu/soya burger or sausage	1 small	1 medium
Healthy fats and oils	1	Nuts and seeds	1 tablespoon	1 heaped tablespoon
		Seed oils, nut oils	2 teaspoons	1 tablespoon
		Oily fish*	60g (2oz)	85g (3oz)

*Oily fish is very rich in essential fats so just one portion a week would more than cover a child's daily needs.

✳ How big is a portion?

The exact portion size depends on the child's age, weight, size and energy needs. In general, younger children need fewer calories than older children so offer them smaller amounts. In the main, be guided by your child's appetite. Remember it is the overall balance of foods that is most important.

How can I make sure my kids get all the nutrients they need everyday?

Here are some simple guidelines to help you plan their daily diet.

Fruit and Vegetables
5+ portions a day
A portion is roughly the amount a child can hold in their hand e.g. 1 apple or banana, 6 strawberries, 2 tablespoons cooked veg.

Why?
Fruit and veg are packed with vitamins and minerals and

other plant nutrients (phytonutrients), which are important for their health and fighting off illnesses.

Make it happen

- O   Whiz fruit with milk or yoghurt to make a smoothie.
- O   Stir chopped veg (e.g. broccoli florets, carrots and colourful peppers) into pasta sauces, soups, curries and hotpots.
- O   Keep frozen and tinned fruits and vegetables on hand for times when fresh produce isn't available. Stock a variety such as tinned beans, peaches (tinned in fruit juice), frozen spinach, cauliflower and peas. Dried fruit also stores well and about 1 tablespoon of raisins or 3 dried apricots matches one portion of fresh fruit.

Are children getting 5 a day?

Children are eating well below the recommended 5 a day for fruit and vegetables. The average intake for girls aged 5 to 15 is 2.6 portions and for boys 2.5 portions, according to the Health Survey for England 2002 report.

Bread, grains and potatoes

6 to 8 portions a day

A portion is 1 slice of bread, half a roll, 3 tablespoons of pasta, rice or breakfast cereal, or 1 (child's) fist-sized potato.

Why?

These foods supply lots of energy. Try to include mostly whole-grain varieties in your child's diet – they contain much higher levels of B-vitamins, iron and fibre.

Make it happen
- ○ Opt for breakfast cereals labelled whole grain, for example Shreddies, Shredded Wheat or Weetabix, or oat-based cereals such as porridge.
- ○ Swap white bread for wholemeal, oatmeal or brown breads.

Calcium-rich Foods
2 portions a day
A portion is 1 cup (200ml) of milk, 25g cheese (size of 4 dice), 1 pot (150g) of yoghurt or fromage frais, or 1 to 2 tablespoons of tinned fish with edible bones (e.g. sardines).

Why?
These foods are rich sources of calcium, which is important for building healthy bones and teeth.

Make it happen
A breakfast of cereal with milk, porridge made with milk, yoghurt and fruit, or a smoothie made with yoghurt or milk gives kids a good part of their daily calcium quota.

Top casseroles, soups, stews, or vegetables with grated cheese. Top baked potatoes with yoghurt or fromage frais.

- ○ It is recommended that children under two should be given full-fat milk because of the extra energy (calories) it provides. Semi-skimmed milk is suitable for the over-twos provided they're eating a varied diet.

✳ Estimated average requirements for energy of children*

Age	Boys (kcal)	Girls (kcal)
4–6 years	1,715	1,545
7–10 years	1,970	1,740

| 11–14 years | 2,220 | 1,845 |
| 15–18 years | 2,755 | 2,110 |

*Department of Health Dietary Reference Values for food energy and nutrients for the United Kingdom (1991) London: HMSO

Protein-rich foods

2 portions a day

A portion is 1 to 2 slices (40–80g) of lean meat, 1 small chicken or turkey breast, 1 small fish fillet, 1 or 2 eggs, 2 to 3 tablespoons of beans or lentils or 1 soya or Quorn 'sausage' or 'burger'.

Why?

These are important sources of protein, which is needed for growth and development. They also provide B-vitamins, iron and zinc.

Make it happen

O   Keep saturated fat in check by opting for leaner cuts of meat, trimming off any visible fat, and removing the skin from chicken or turkey.

O   Limit processed meats (burgers, sausages and nuggets) to once a week, because they contain a lot of saturated fat and salt.

O   Even if your family are not vegetarian, try to introduce some vegetable protein foods into your children's diet. Try beans and lentils in soups, salads, curries, Bolognese sauce, stews, chilli and shepherd's pie. These foods provide a unique type of fibre that's particularly beneficial for the digestive system, as well as lots of important plant nutrients not found in animal proteins.

Are organic meat and milk healthier?

Organic meat may be regarded as healthier because it contains none of the antibiotics and hormones routinely used in conventional farming, and many experts are concerned about the effects these may have on humans. Some believe that the accumulation of antibiotics from eating meat lowers people's immunity and makes it more difficult to fight infections with regular antibiotics. Many people also choose organic milk for the same reasons. It is also more nutritious: Newcastle researchers found that organic milk contains 50 per cent more vitamin E and 68 per cent more omega-3s than other milk, according to a 2006 study by the Institute of Environmental and Grasslands Research.

Healthy fats and oils

1 to 2 portions a day

A portion is 1 to 2 tablespoons of nuts or seeds, 1 tablespoon of olive oil or other seed/nut oils, half an avocado or one (140g) portion of oily fish once a week.

Why?

These foods are excellent sources of essential fats, especially the omega-3 fats, important for maintaining healthy brain, eye and nerve function.

Make it happen

O   Include at least one portion (140g) of oily fish per week – try tinned sardines on toast or a wrap filled with tinned salmon and lettuce.

○ Nuts and seeds are perfect for snacks but you can also add them to breakfast cereal, yoghurt, salads and stir-fries.

When can children be given nuts?

It is recommended that young children under three years old with a family history of allergy should not be given peanuts in any form. But children with no allergy history can be given peanuts and other nut products after the age of one. Nuts can cause serious allergies in a small proportion of children and peanuts seem to cause the worst reaction. Your child is more likely to be affected if you or another family member suffers from asthma, eczema or hay fever. Whole nuts should not be given to children under five years old because of the risk of choking, but they can be used finely ground or as peanut butter.

Why is my child a fussy eater?

Most children go through phases of fussy eating. Toddlers quickly realise that food is one area where they have control. Refusing a particular food is a way of asserting their independence and gaining attention. The more firmly they reject a particular food, the more attention they get and a vicious circle is soon established. Mealtimes then present the perfect opportunity to test the boundaries. Some children are very good at using food to wind up their parents. The more firmly they refuse to finish their plate at mealtimes, the more attention they get. They know that refusing food results in attention.

Fussy eating may be linked to a child's personality. If they are strongly independent, they are more likely to want to gain control of their eating environment.

How should I deal with fussy eating?

Faddy eating habits can persist for many years – and the earlier you tackle the issue, the better. The first thing to remember is that children don't voluntarily starve themselves: they're programmed for survival! As long as there's food available, children will make sure they get enough.

Try these solutions for fussy eaters:

Get them in the kitchen: Encourage your children to help with the shopping and preparing meals. This will increase their interest in the food, and they'll be more likely to eat the meal if they've been involved in making it.

Be a good role model: Children learn by example so let them see that you enjoy eating healthy meals. They're more likely to eat foods that they've seen you eat, too. Have meals together whenever possible – ideally once a day, otherwise at least once a week – and show them you enjoy trying new tastes. Serve your children the same food as everyone else.

Build up their appetite: Ensure they've taken plenty of fresh air and exercise; they do wonders for the appetite. It's amazing how less fussy children become if they are really hungry!

Let children serve themselves: Put the food in dishes in the centre of the table so everyone can serve himself or herself. By the age of four most children can judge how much they can eat. You'll also be helping them become more socially aware and independent, allowing them to make their own choices and take responsibility for their actions.

Think small: Even if the portion seems ridiculously tiny to you, it's better that your child eats a small amount of everything than nothing at all. A big pile of food on the plate can be off-putting for young children. As a rule of thumb, the younger the child, the smaller the pieces of food – try tiny broccoli florets, small squares of toast or super-thin apple slices.

Keep mealtimes happy: Meals should be enjoyable. Don't discuss eating behaviour, negative food or family issues at mealtimes. Try to achieve a relaxed atmosphere – keep conversation light and fun.

Play with food: You can encourage fussy eaters, especially younger children, to eat good food by presenting it imaginatively. Arrange food in simple shapes, say a circle, a star, a face or a train, or try playing games – such as the train (broccoli) going into the tunnel (mouth)!

Keep it simple: Offer simple and plain foods, such as baked potatoes, cheese and carrots. Fussy eaters prefer to see exactly what they're eating. They can be put off if they're presented with lots of different foods on their plate, or dishes where they can't identify the component foods.

Don't get cross: If your child refuses the meal or certain foods, keep your temper. Explain that you expect them to try it and don't offer an alternative. You need to be patient but persistent – not easy, I know, especially when you've spent time preparing a meal. Refusing food loses its appeal if you don't react.

Don't force-feed: You can't make a child eat – he or she will react to your concern and will be even less likely to eat the food. Most adults have bad memories of being made to eat a particular food as a child – remember school dinners? – and then hating it ever since!

Don't bargain with food: It's tempting to say – 'no pudding unless you've eaten your vegetables'. But never promise children a favourite food or dessert only when they've finished their main course – this will only reinforce the dislike of the refused food and make the other food seem more special. It's reasonable to expect them to try everything, so you could ask them to have, say, two sprouts as a compromise. This will seem less daunting.

Keep trying! If a food is rejected, it doesn't mean they'll never eat it. Children's tastes do change over time. Keep reintroducing those foods they reject, maybe once a fortnight or once a month, and don't make a fuss. It can take up to eight to ten attempts to get a child to eat a new food. Don't reinforce their dislike of a particular food by telling everyone else that your child won't eat, say, tomatoes, or whatever. He'll be even less likely to try it again.

Give them options: Encourage children to select their own food but from within a limited choice, e.g. 'Would you like beans or peas with that?' rather than 'Would you like vegetables?'

Set a time limit: If they refuse to eat the meal within, say, thirty minutes, remove it without fuss and don't offer any other food until next mealtime. Be consistent and remember that they won't become malnourished straight away.

Be strict with snacks: If they don't eat their meal, don't let them fill up on snacks later. Eating between meals will simply take away their appetites for more nutritious foods at mealtimes, and perpetuate their taste for those salty, sugary processed foods. If they're genuinely hungry, offer only nutritious food – such as fruit, cheese, yoghurt or nuts.

Can fussy eating run in families?

Fussy eating isn't inherited but children's food likes and dislikes are certainly influenced by their parents' eating habits. According to a 2002 US study, this occurs as early as the age of two. If the mother doesn't like a food, she is less likely to offer it to her children. But it's worth making the effort to introduce your children to new tastes even if you aren't keen on the food yourself – kids are more likely to accept new foods early on, before the age of eight.

Chapter 2

Weight Loss

I will never be a thin girl. I tend to put on a bit of weight over the winter, like a plump little squirrel. I seem to gain weight very easily, especially if I don't exercise. I did my back in recently and couldn't do proper exercise for three weeks, and I went up a dress size in that time.

For me, the key to maintaining a healthy weight is all about combining healthy eating with exercise. I don't weigh myself, but rather I use how I feel in my clothes as an indication of whether I need to lose some weight.

If you're trying to lose weight, do make sure you combine healthy eating with exercise. You will lose weight more easily and you will have so much more energy. The simplest thing is to get up off your bottom and go for a walk a few times a week, starting off slowly and then building up your pace and distance.

The worrying news is that obesity rates in the UK have almost quadrupled in the last twenty-five years. Around eight million people (22 per cent) in the UK were obese in 2008. And obesity has been linked to a whole host of serious illnesses.

In this chapter, you learn the facts about why we

gain and lose weight, whether there is any value in the latest celebrity diets, plus plenty of handy and simple-to-follow tips if you need to lose weight.

❄️

What is the difference between 'obesity' and 'overweight'?

Obesity is defined as a level of body fat which is harmful to health. It can be measured by comparing your body mass index (BMI, see 'What is my BMI?' below) with the population average. People with a BMI above 25 are 'overweight'; those above 30 are 'obese'.

What is my BMI?

Your 'body mass index' or BMI is a measure of body fat based on height and weight. The BMI is calculated by dividing your weight (kg) by the square of your height (m^2).

For example, if your weight is 60kg and height 1.7m, your BMI is:

60 ÷ (1.7 x 1.7) = 21

Your goal should be to maintain your BMI between 18.5 and 24.9. You can calculate your BMI from the chart on page 87. First select your height, then select your weight. Select the nearest value to your own if they are not displayed in the chart. Your Body Mass Index will be listed at the top and bottom of the BMI chart.

Normal weight (18.5–24.9), Overweight (25–29.9), Obesity (30+)

BMI	19	20	21	22	23	24	25	26	27	28	29	30	31	32	33	34	35
Height cm (m)	Body Weight (kilograms)																
147cm (1.47m)	41	44	45	48	50	52	54	56	59	61	63	65	67	69	72	73	76
150cm (1.50m)	43	45	47	49	52	54	56	58	60	63	65	67	69	72	74	76	78
152cm (1.52m)	44	46	49	51	54	56	58	60	63	65	67	69	72	74	76	79	81
155cm (1.55m)	45	48	50	53	55	57	60	62	65	67	69	72	74	77	79	82	84
157cm (1.57m)	47	49	52	54	57	59	62	64	67	69	72	74	77	79	82	84	87
160cm (1.60m)	49	51	54	56	59	61	64	66	69	72	74	77	79	82	84	87	89
163cm (1.63m)	50	53	55	58	61	64	66	68	71	74	77	79	82	84	87	89	93
165cm (1.65m)	52	54	57	60	63	65	68	71	73	76	79	82	84	87	90	93	95
168cm (1.68m)	54	56	59	62	64	67	70	73	76	78	81	84	87	90	93	95	98
170cm (1.70m)	55	57	61	64	66	69	72	75	78	81	84	87	90	93	96	98	101
172cm (1.72m)	57	59	63	65	68	72	74	78	80	83	86	89	92	95	98	101	104
175cm (1.75m)	58	61	64	68	70	73	77	80	83	86	89	92	95	98	101	104	107
178cm (1.78m)	60	63	66	69	73	76	79	82	85	88	92	95	98	101	104	107	110
180cm (1.80m)	62	65	68	71	75	78	81	84	88	91	94	98	101	104	107	110	113
183cm (1.83m)	64	67	70	73	77	80	83	87	90	93	97	100	103	107	110	113	117
185cm (1.85m)	65	68	72	75	79	83	86	89	93	96	99	103	107	110	113	117	120
188cm (1.88m)	67	70	74	78	81	84	88	92	95	99	102	106	109	113	116	120	123
191cm (1.91m)	69	73	76	80	83	87	91	94	98	102	105	109	112	116	120	123	127
193cm (1.93m)	71	74	78	82	86	89	93	97	100	104	108	112	115	119	123	127	130
BMI	19	20	21	22	23	24	25	26	27	28	29	30	31	32	33	34	35

Aren't there better ways of measuring fatness?

The BMI is a useful method but it doesn't take into account where fat is stored in your body. This is important because 'apple'-shaped people (with most of their fat stored around the abdomen) are more at risk of developing obesity-related diseases such as type 2 diabetes, high blood pressure and heart disease, than 'pear' shapes who have most fat on their hips. The BMI also does not allow for how much muscle you have.

Try the following tests to find out your health risk:

1. Measure your waist: This tells you roughly the amount of fat you carry in your abdomen and is regarded as more accurate than BMI in predicting type 2 diabetes risk. For women, if your waist measures more than 80cm (32 inches), or for men, more than 94cm (37 inches), then you need to lose weight.
2. Divide your waist measurement by your hip measurement: This will tell you whether you are an 'apple' or a 'pear'. If the figure is greater than 0.85 for women or 0.95 for men, you are an apple and more at risk from diseases linked to obesity.

How can fat around my waist be a health risk?

A high waist measurement indicates excess visceral fat, the unseen fat in your abdominal cavity around your internal organs. The problem with this type of fat is that it doesn't just sit there. It actively alters the body's normal hormonal and chemical balances, pumping out sex hormones, insulin and inflammatory and clot-producing compounds. These changes increase levels of 'bad' LDL cholesterol, and also send signals that may cause cancer to grow. So a man with a 'beer belly' but slim limbs may be at greater risk of heart disease, diabetes and cancer than a pear-shaped person with the same BMI but less visceral fat.

I'm not ill now so is it really unhealthy to be overweight?

Statistically, being overweight increases your risk of developing a wide range of health problems including:

- diabetes
- high blood pressure and high blood cholesterol
- heart disease
- a number of cancers, including breast, womb, kidney, colon and prostate
- arthritis
- period problems
- infertility
- miscarriage, illness in pregnancy, and difficulty in labour
- indigestion
- gallstones
- snoring and sleep apnoea

Obese women are nearly thirteen times more likely to develop diabetes than women of normal weight, more than four times as likely to suffer high blood pressure and three times as likely to develop cancer of the colon. Obese men are more than five times as likely to develop diabetes as those of normal weight, more than twice as likely to suffer high blood pressure and about twice as likely to develop osteoarthritis.

Overweight and physical inactivity together account for about a third of all premature deaths, two thirds of deaths from cardiovascular disease, and a fifth of deaths from cancer among non-smokers, according to a 2005 US study.

Are overweight kids at risk of health problems too?

Yes. Being overweight affects children psychologically and physically. Overweight children are more likely to be teased, bullied and suffer from low self-esteem and self-worth. A

2006 study of more than 8,000 seven-year olds carried out by University College London found that obese children were 50 per cent more likely to be bullied than average-weight classmates.

Overweight children are more likely to develop bone and joint problems, breathing problems and asthma, high blood pressure, high blood cholesterol, type 2 diabetes, artery damage during their teens and early adulthood, and heart disease and stroke in later life. According to a 2007 study at Washington University, US, children who are obese show early signs of heart disease similar to obese adults with heart disease. A 2005 study at St George's Medical School, London, found that carrying even a small amount of excess fat in your early teens can lead to cardiovascular disease. Obese children are also up to 20 per cent more likely to develop cancer as adults, according to a 2004 statement from the National Obesity Forum. Most seriously overweight children are likely to grow up to become fat adults. Children who are obese in their teens are twice as likely to die by age fifty.

❊ Is your child overweight?

It is more difficult to gauge whether children are overweight or obese than adults because they are growing anyway, and do so at different rates. The fit of a child's clothes is a rough measure. If clothes for their age are right for their height but too tight around the waist, they could be overweight. You can check your child's weight using Body Mass Index (BMI) charts for children. They show what a healthy BMI would be for a particular age. To calculate your child's BMI divide their weight in kg by their height in metres squared (e.g. if a child weighs 35kg and is 1.25m tall, their BMI would be 22.4).

To calculate your child's BMI, and for an interpretation of the results, go to www.weightconcern.org.uk or check the chart below.

BMIs for overweight or obese children

Age	Overweight		Obese	
	Boys	Girls	Boys	Girls
5	17.4	17.1	19.3	19.2
6	17.6	17.3	19.8	19.7
7	17.9	17.8	20.6	20.5
8	18.4	18.3	21.6	21.6
9	19.1	19.1	22.8	22.8
10	19.8	19.9	24.0	24.1
11	20.6	20.7	25.1	25.4
12	21.2	21.7	26.0	26.7
13	21.9	22.6	26.8	27.8

Why do I gain weight easily while others remain slim?

People who generally have little problem controlling their weight seem to have a precisely tuned appetite, while people who struggle to control their weight may be less sensitive to their body's signals of fullness. There's no single explanation – scientists believe a number of factors working together cause obesity. Your genetic make-up, prenatal development, lifestyle and environment all have a role to play. But, whatever the contributory factors, you will deposit fat on your body if you eat more energy than you use.

Can my genes make me fat?

Lots of people like to blame their weight problems on their genes! Indeed, fatness often appears to run families – if you're overweight chances are one or both of your parents are too. Children with two obese parents have a 70 per cent risk of becoming obese, compared with 20 per cent in children with two lean parents. Studies with identical twins suggest that genes may account for up to 25 per cent of your overweight. Scientists have identified several genes that influence body shape, fat distribution around the body, your appetite, as well as how fast or slow you burn the calories you eat.

But diet, activity and other lifestyle habits also 'run in families' – they have nothing to do with genes. These are behaviours children pick up from their parents and carry into adulthood and then pass down to their children. If your family has a habit of eating high-fat food and sitting around, that probably explains the 'family fat'. If, on the other hand, your family is physically active and do lots of sports, you may all be slim and fit.

You cannot change your genes but you can change your eating and activity habits. Even if the genes are stacked against you, you can be slim; you may just have to eat a little less than others or exercise a bit more.

Is it true that a mother's diet can put her baby on the path to obesity?

Yes, we always say 'you are what you eat' but there's mounting evidence that 'you are what your mother ate'. A 2005 US study found that children born to women who put on excess weight during pregnancy were more likely to become overweight themselves. According to a 2007 UK study, mothers who ate a diet of junk food during pregnancy and breast-feeding are more likely to have overweight babies with a preference for junk food. In other words, a craving for junk food may begin in the womb. In 2008, the same London-based researchers found that these babies were more likely to develop weight problems and health problems in later life.

Can a baby's diet increase their risk of obesity later on?

Several studies over the last few years have suggested that what you ate as a baby could make you more or less prone to obesity as you get older. In 2007, German researchers revealed that babies who had a relatively higher protein intake (particularly from dairy foods) around the age of twelve months were more likely to have a higher BMI and body-fat percentage in later years. It is thought that this may be due to the sudden switch from mother's milk (high fat, low protein) to a typical weaning diet, which is lower in fat but high in dairy protein. Whilst a certain amount of protein is essential for growth, too much seems to encourage the growth of fat cells and increase fat storage. In practical terms, babies over six months should have a varied diet but not be overfed protein-rich foods such as dairy foods.

What's to blame then – too much food or lack of exercise?

Both, probably. Some experts prefer to blame our couch-potato lifestyle for the rise in obesity, citing the fact that people in the 1950s ate more calories than people today but were much slimmer because their daily lives involved far more physical activity. Indeed, many studies show that obese people tend to live sedentary lifestyles and that obese children prefer sedentary activities to physical ones, if given the option. On the other hand, a 2008 study by a team at Peninsula Medical School in Plymouth suggests that the obesity epidemic is caused more by eating too much than how much activity you do. They found that children who did more exercise were healthier, but the amount of activity they did had no effect on how fat they were. What's clear is that you have to match your food intake (calories in) with your lifestyle and activity (calories out).

Why can some people eat whatever they want without gaining weight?

Some people may appear to eat whatever they want, but the truth is they don't, in fact, overeat nor do they eat as much as overweight people. Naturally slim people seem to have an inborn ability to regulate their calorie intake. They're able to sense when they have had enough to eat and don't overstep the mark. Scientists at Pennsylvania State University in the US call this an in-built calorie counter. It's controlled by a gene, which is responsible for giving the brain the message, 'You're full so stop eating' or 'You need to increase your activity so exercise more'. That way they don't get fat.

✳ How our shapes have changed

According to a 2007 study at University College London, the average British woman weighs 66kg (10st 5lb) and her vital statistics are 39–34–41: a far cry from those of the average woman in the 1950s whose waist was 27 inches and whose hips and bust were both 34 inches. The typical British man weighs 80kg (12½ stones) and his waist has expanded from 30 inches in the 1950s to 37 inches.

Is obesity 'contagious'?

Possibly, depending on the company you keep. Having friends and family who are overweight raises your risk of being overweight too, according to a 2007 US study published in the *New England Journal of Medicine*. The data on more than 12,000 people over 32 years suggests the risk increases by 57 per cent if a friend is obese, by 40 per cent if a sibling is obese and 37 per cent if a spouse is.

Of course, obesity isn't contagious in a physical sense, but having overweight family or friends changes your norms about what counts as an appropriate body size. It's easy to think that it is OK to be bigger when those around you are bigger.

Why am I fat when I hardly eat a thing?

Do you really eat as little as you think you do? A US study found that women typically reported eating 400 fewer calories per day than they actually ate. One in four women under-reported by more than 800 calories. The more overweight the women were, the more calories they under-reported. Try measuring your food and keeping a food diary to see exactly what you eat and where your downfalls lie. Choose smaller portions of calorie-dense foods (desserts, cheese, margarine) and fill up with foods that have a low calorie density (fruit, vegetables, salad).

I often have my main meal late in the evening – is this bad for me?

Eating a big meal in the evening, especially just before going to bed, puts a strain on the digestive organs and saps your energy. You risk waking up feeling sluggish the next morning. Instead, keep your energy levels up by eating small meals and snacks through the day, while reducing the size of your evening meal.

Is it true that fat people have a slower metabolism than slim people?

No. In fact the opposite is true! The heavier you are, the higher your metabolic rate. It's a basic law of physics – larger people need more energy to pump the blood around the body and to keep moving. Just as bigger cars use more fuel than small cars, so bigger people use more energy than small people. The hard truth is slim people don't burn up calories any quicker – they just don't consume as many.

What's my metabolic rate?

Your *metabolic rate* is the rate at which your body burns calories. Your *basal metabolic rate* (BMR) is the rate at which you burn calories at rest on essential body functions, such as breathing and blood circulation. It accounts for 60 to 75 per cent of calories burned daily.

BMR uses roughly 22 calories for every kilo of a woman's weight and 24 calories per kilo of a man's weight.

For women: BMR (calories) = weight in kg x 22
For men: BMR (calories) = weight in kg x 24

For example, for a 60kg woman: BMR = 60 x 22= 1,320 calories

What makes my metabolic rate high or low?

The most important factor is your weight. In general, the more you weigh, the higher your BMR. Muscular people also have a higher BMR – muscle burns about three times more calories than fat. Genetics is also important – some people are born with a more 'revved up' metabolism than others.

Does my metabolism slow down with age?

It will slow down unless you exercise regularly. You'll lose around 0.25kg (½lb) of muscle every year after your late twenties. And as you lose muscle, your BMR drops about 2 per cent each decade so your body burns fewer calories. You can combat age-related muscle loss with twice-weekly weight training.

How can I boost my metabolism?

Here are five things you can do to boost your metabolism and burn more calories:

Get moving: During the hour or two after vigorous exercise you continue burning calories faster than normal, as your body replenishes its energy reserves and repairs muscle tissue. The longer and more intense the workout, the greater will be this 'after-burn'. And repeated short bursts of high intensity activity revs the metabolism and burns more fat according to study at the University of New South Wales.

Tone up: To increase your metabolic rate in the long term you have to add muscle.

A 1997 study at the University of Limburg found that twice-weekly weights workout increased metabolic rate by 10 per cent on average. Muscle burns more calories than fat so the more muscle you have the greater your daily calorie burn. Select a weight that allows you to just complete eight to twelve repetitions (if you can do more, up the weight) – this will have a bigger effect on your metabolic rate than using lighter weights.

Eat small meals often through the day: Eating small regular meals keeps your metabolism ticking over and is a much better way to burn off calories than, say, one meal a day. Plan three meals and two or three snacks a day, spacing them at two- to three-hour intervals. Your metabolism is boosted by about 10 per cent for two to three hours after you eat. Avoid skipping meals or leaving more than five hours between meals.

Get enough protein: While eating anything raises your metabolic rate, protein boosts it the most. Up to 20 per cent of such a meal's calories may be burned off as heat, according to a study published in the *American Journal of Clinical Nutrition*. Protein is also the most satisfying nutrient, so helps stop you overeating.

Eat a healthy breakfast: Your metabolic rate slows dramatically during sleep and you burn fewer calories per hour as a result. Breakfast kick-starts your metabolism and allows you the whole day to burn up those calories. A combination of carbohydrate and protein (say, porridge made with milk) will give you sustained energy.

Is breakfast really the most important meal of the day?

It's important to eat either first thing in the morning, or at least within a couple of hours of waking. Breakfast stabilises blood-sugar levels, which regulates your energy levels. It also reduces the risk of overeating later in the day, as you'll have satisfied your hunger. Keep your senses sharp by eating a low GI breakfast of porridge or a fruit and yoghurt smoothie. Researchers at Reading University found that people who eat a low GI breakfast perform better at mental tasks than those eating a sugary breakfast.

What's the secret to long-term successful weight loss?

The only way to lose weight is to take in fewer calories than your body needs for basic functions and daily activities. If you eat 3,500 more calories than you need, they will be stored and add half a kilo (1lb) to your weight. On the other hand, burn 3,500 more calories than you eat and you'll lose half a kilo (1lb). This isn't as daunting as it seems. Aim to create a daily calorie deficit of 500 calories by eating a little less and being more active. For example, you could cut out a packet of crisps and a glass of wine to save 300 calories; and walk an extra 40 minutes to burn 200 calories. Over a week, this will result in a calorie deficit of 3,500 and a weight loss of half a kilo (1lb).

To get an idea of how many calories you should be eating every day, use the calculator on www.healthstatus.com.

Alternatively, you can estimate your daily calorie needs using the formulae on page 96.

☀ Why diets don't work long-term

Diets may help people to lose weight, but the problem is keeping it off. Most people who lose weight on a diet put it on again. Only 5 per cent of obese people manage to keep their weight down. In 2007 researchers at the University of California reviewed thirty-one previous studies and found that during the first six months of a diet people typically lost between 5 and 10 per cent of their weight, but within five years two out of three put more weight on than they had lost. Most would have been better off not going on the diet at all.

How fast can I lose weight?

Experts agree between half and one kilo (1–2lb) per week is a healthy and effective rate of weight loss. A loss of more than one kilo (2lb) per week means you could be losing muscle.

Will cutting more calories help me lose weight faster?

Going on a strict diet may cause the pounds to drop off but can make you feel lethargic and weak. Worse, your body can end up hoarding instead of burning fat. A sudden drop in calories tells your body to conserve energy, as starvation might be imminent. Your body goes into survival mode and the rate at which you burn energy slows down. Your body adapts to survive on a lower calorie intake, which means

Weight Loss 99

that when you stop dieting, you're likely to put the weight back on. To compensate for the low calorie intake, your body will start to break down muscle tissue for fuel. So, you can end up losing muscle as well as fat. You should not cut your current calorie intake by more than 15 per cent.

What is a healthy body-fat percentage?

Scientists recommend body-fat levels between 18 and 25 per cent for women and 13 to 18 per cent for men. These ranges are associated with the lowest health risk in population studies.

According to 2008 US research, if your body-fat percentage is more than 30 per cent (for women) or more than 20 per cent (for men) yet your BMI is 'normal' then you are just as unhealthy as those considered obese. It means you're carrying too much fat around your organs, which puts you at risk of diabetes and heart disease. Measuring your body-fat percentage using skinfold callipers (ideally by a health or fitness professional) or bioelectrical impedance (e.g. body composition scales) will tell you how much of your body is lean muscle and how much is fat.

✳ How to set yourself a good goal

A good goal should be made up of five elements:

Personal: You have to believe in and truly want to achieve your goal, e.g. 'I know that losing weight will allow me to fit into my clothes more comfortably and make me feel more confident, so I will begin to eat more healthily and take more exercise.'

Specific: You need to clearly define what you want to achieve, prioritise steps, organise plans and establish a timescale for reaching your goal, e.g. 'I will limit myself to one chocolate bar once a week, on Saturdays, and eat three portions of fruit each day in place of biscuits.'

Realistic: Your goal has to be realistic and attainable for your body shape and lifestyle, e.g. 'I will lose three kilos in six weeks.'

Measurable: You need to state how you will know when you've reached your goal. So you should state your goals in terms of weight loss, body measurements or body-fat percentage, e.g. 'I will lose half a kilo each week.' Keeping a food diary and training log will help you monitor your progress and allow you to see whether you met the goal.

Agreed: Agree your goal with someone else and write it down. This signals a commitment to change and makes it more likely that you will achieve your goal.

Time-scaled: You need a plan of action with deadlines. It's helpful to break down your long-term goal into several short-term goals that can be achieved weekly and monthly.

Reward yourself: Rewarding yourself when you have reached a goal helps you stay motivated and focused on reaching your goals. Rewards can be something simple like a star for reaching a weekly target or something tangible like a new pair of shoes, a CD, a theatre trip or a beauty treatment.

Why do experts tell dieters to keep a food diary?

Keeping a food diary will give you a much clearer idea of what you are really eating and where your calories are coming from. Write down everything that passes your lips for three days (or longer if you can manage it), noting the portion weights and sizes. Try to be as accurate as possible, recording the weights of everything and remembering to write down every snack and every drink. Be as honest as possible – that handful of crisps, those biscuits with your tea, that glass of wine after work. You may be surprised how many calories you eat or how often you nibble.

How can I stop feeling hungry every time I want to lose weight?

To lose weight you need to be able to choose foods that satisfy your appetite for the longest time yet provide relatively few calories. The more satiated you feel after a meal the less food you will eat at the next one and the longer you will keep hunger at bay. To feel full on fewer calories, eat mostly foods with a low calorie density – in other words, foods that contain relatively few calories per gram (see table page 103). These foods provide maximum filling power for fewest calories, and thus help control your appetite and stave off hunger pangs. Reducing the amount of fat you eat lowers the energy density of your diet. It means you can eat bigger portions for the same or even fewer calories. Substitute reduced-fat or low-fat versions for high-fat foods (e.g. skimmed instead of whole milk). Use lower-fat cooking methods (e.g. grilling instead of frying).

What is the calorie density of foods?

This tells you how many calories are in each gram of a particular food. To calculate a food's calorie density, divide the number of calories in a serving by its weight in grams.

Calorie density = calories (per portion) ÷ grams (per portion)

For example, the calorie density of a 29g cereal bar providing 124 calories is:

Calorie density = 124 ÷ 29 = 4.28

The calorie density of foods

Very low energy density (0–0.6) Eat satisfying portions	Most fruits (e.g. strawberries, apples, oranges), non-starchy vegetables (e.g. carrots, broccoli), salad vegetables (e.g. lettuce, cucumber), skimmed milk, clear soups, fat-free or plain yoghurt
Low energy density (0.6–1.5) Eat satisfying or moderate portions	Bananas, starchy vegetables (e.g. sweet corn, potatoes), low-fat plain/fruit yoghurt, pulses (beans, lentils and peas), pasta, rice and other cooked grains, breakfast cereals with low-fat milk
Medium energy density (1.5–4.0) Eat moderate or small portions	Meat, poultry, cheeses, eggs, pizza, chips (fries), raisins, salad dressings, bread, ice cream, cake
High energy density (4.0–9.0) Eat small portions or substitute low-fat versions	Crackers, crisps, chocolate, sweets, croissants, biscuits, cereal bars, nuts, butter and oils

Will lots of fibre make me lose more weight?

Fibre expands in the gut, makes you feel full and helps stop you overeating. It also helps to satisfy your hunger by slowing the rate that foods pass through your digestive system and stabilising blood-sugar levels. Studies have shown that people who increased their fibre intake for four months ate fewer calories and lost an average of five pounds– with no dieting! Try replacing half of your usual portion of meat or pasta dish with vegetables. That way you won't feel like you're eating less. Add extra vegetables to sauces, soups and stews as 'stealth' vegetables. Not only will they lower the calorie content of the portion you eat, they will also boost the nutritional content of the meal.

Will using a smaller plate make me eat less?

Yes, the smaller the portion, the less you eat! In a 2005 experiment at Cornell University in the US, volunteers were given either a medium (120g) or large (240g) box of popcorn while watching a film. The people who were given the large boxes ate 45 per cent more than those given the medium boxes – 100 more calories, to be exact. Even if the popcorn was stale, the volunteers still ate 30 per cent more. Drinking from a bigger cup also makes you drink more and consume more calories. A 2006 study at Penn State University found that when volunteers were given a larger serving of drink with a meal, they drank 50 per cent more and consumed up to 25 per cent more calories.

I keep reading about 'satiety' and 'SI' – can this help me lose weight?

Satiety is a measure of how long the consumption of a particular food will stop you feeling hungry again.

The satiety index (SI), developed by Australian scientists in 1995, ranks different foods on their ability to produce satiety. Foods high on the satiety index list, such as potatoes and porridge, keep hunger pangs at bay longer while those low on the scale, such as cakes and croissants, are more likely to have you reaching for the cookie jar sooner.

To feel full longer, select mostly foods with an SI greater than 100.

The satiety index

All are compared to white bread (100).

Croissant	47
Cake	65
Doughnuts	68
Mars bar	70
Peanuts	84
Yoghurt	88
Ice cream	96
Muesli	100
White bread	100
Sustain cereal	112
French fries	116
Special K	116
Bananas	118
Corn flakes	118
Jelly beans	118
White pasta	119
Cookies	120
Crackers	127
Brown rice	132
Lentils	133
White rice	138
Cheese	146
Eggs	150
All-Bran	151
Grain bread	154
Popcorn	154
Wholemeal bread	157
Grapes	162
Baked beans	168
Beef	176
Whole-wheat pasta	188
Apples	197
Oranges	202
Porridge	209
White fish	225
Potatoes	323

↑ Less satisfying

↓ More satisfying

It's difficult to know what is the right portion. How can I work out how much I should be eating?

Here is a guide to help you estimate portion sizes:

One cupped hand = 1 portion (80g) of vegetables

Two cupped hands = 1 portion (80g) of salad

Size of a tennis ball = 1 portion (80g) of fruit, e.g. apple, peach

One cupped hand = 1 portion (80g) of berries or chopped fruit

Size of a tennis ball = 1 portion of potatoes (150g)

Two cupped hands = 1 portion (40g) of breakfast cereal flakes

One small cupped hand = 1 portion (25g) of nuts or seeds

Deck of cards = 1 portion (85g) of cooked meat or fish

Size of 4 dice = 1 portion (25g) of cheese

One generous cupped hand = 1 portion (40g dry weight) of pasta

One cupped hand = 1 portion (30g) of rice

200ml glass or cup = 1 portion of milk or fruit juice

✳ The benefits of exercise

Increasing the amount of physical activity you do will not only speed weight loss but will also significantly lower your risk of heart disease, stroke, diabetes and cancer. Regular exercise helps reduce blood pressure and blood-cholesterol levels, strengthens your muscles and bones, reduces stress and improves psychological wellbeing.

How much exercise do I need to do for weight loss?

To keep your heart healthy, experts recommend spending thirty minutes doing some kind of activity that makes you breathe faster and your heart beat faster on at least five days a week. Three ten-minute sessions of exercise produce the same fitness results as one thirty-minute session. But, to *lose weight*, you should aim for at least sixty minutes moderate cardiovascular exercise most days of the week, according to government guidelines.

Which type of exercise produces the fastest weight loss?

Cardiovascular activities such as walking or swimming at an easy pace burn fat but you will need to do them for long periods to burn significant calories and lose weight. Step up the intensity and you'll shed pounds faster. In a study at the University of Wisconsin, women who cycled strenuously for twenty-five minutes daily lost the same amount of body fat as those who cycled at a more leisurely pace for fifty minutes daily.

But for fastest weight loss, do interval training, alternating short bursts of intense activity with lower intensity periods, during which you recover. A study at Quebec University found that this type of exercise burned three and a half times more body fat than steady-state, moderate-intensity exercise. Try one or two minutes of high-intensity alternating with two minutes of recovery. For example, if you're swimming, try alternating easy-paced lengths with some fast lengths.

Doesn't exercise make you hungrier?

No. Regular exercise actually improves appetite control so you'll find it easier to control your weight. In fact, a 2008 study from the University of Michigan, US, found that normal-weight women reported feeling less hungry after exercise, whereas obese women did not. The good news is that as you continue exercising and losing weight, you'll find it easier to control your appetite.

Does exercising on an empty stomach burn more fat?

If fat loss is your goal, the best time to do cardiovascular exercise is on an empty stomach when insulin levels are low. This encourages the muscles to burn fat rather than carbohydrate. You won't necessarily burn more calories but more of the calories you do burn will come from fat. Over time, this may lead to speedier fat loss. But if fitness is your goal, eat a light snack one to two hours before exercising. The resulting rise in blood-sugar levels will help you exercise longer and so you will burn more calories.

What are the best tips for losing weight?

Listen to your hunger signals

Make an effort to differentiate between true hunger and emotional hunger. Try to gauge how much food your body really needs and then eat the amount that is right for you. This may take practice but you will soon become attuned to your body's needs and learn to eat appropriate portions of food.

Thirsty or hungry?

Many people confuse thirst with hunger. Both sensations are generated in the same part of the brain, the satiety centre, to indicate the brain's satiety needs. If you don't recognise the sensation of thirst, you may assume that you are hungry, so you eat instead of drinking water. Next time you're feeling peckish, drink a glass of water and wait ten minutes to see if you are still hungry.

Keep temptation out of the way

It may sound obvious, but if you want to avoid the temptation of diet-wrecking snacks, don't bring them into your house. Although you may think you can control your consumption, it's a lot easier if the only things in the kitchen are fruit and vegetables, rather than crisps and biscuits.

Slow down

Eating your food slowly and in a relaxed state of mind will curb your desire to eat more than you need. According to research at the University of Florida, eating quickly means the satiety centre in the brain doesn't receive the right signals and explains why you may feel hungrier sooner. Cut your food into smaller pieces, chew each mouthful thoroughly and don't load your fork with more food before swallowing the previous mouthful. Try putting down your knife and fork between mouthfuls.

If you eat too fast you won't be able to digest your food properly. The digestive process starts in the mouth and continues in the stomach – if food isn't broken down thoroughly your body won't be able to absorb the nutrients it needs for long-term energy.

Get into a routine

Make an effort to schedule regular meals that fit around your hunger, not your daily commitments. Leading a busy, stressful life often causes your eating patterns to become haphazard. The result is you end up eating when you're not hungry. You can lose the ability to make the connection between true hunger and eating, and end up overeating.

Eat a healthy breakfast

People who skip breakfast are more likely to overeat later in the day and pile on unwanted pounds, according to a 2008 study from Venezuela. Researchers found that women who ate most of their calories early in the day lost 39lb over 8 months, while those who followed a conventional diet lost only 10lb. When you start your day off with a healthy filling breakfast, you dramatically increase your chances of eating healthily throughout the day. A big breakfast also helps control your appetite and cravings for snacks.

Put leftovers out of sight
To avoid overeating at mealtimes, serve your portion and then put any leftovers out of sight. If you don't have the dish on the table in front of you there will be less temptation to keep refilling your plate. Get into the habit of freezing leftovers or putting them in the fridge immediately, away from temptation.

Don't be fooled by 'diet' labels
If you eat food that looks like it should be high calorie or high fat but actually isn't, your body will soon cotton on. Experiments show that once it realises a food's appearance and taste promises don't match up its calorie properties your body adjusts your hunger response so you no longer feel satisfied eating that food. The calorie savings of many low-fat foods are often small anyway – as sugar replaces most of the fat reduction. Studies show that people who consume large quantities of diet drinks have the highest intake of calories.

Eat without distractions
When you're not concentrating on your meal it's harder to listen to your body and recognise when you are full. A study by French researchers measured how much women ate for lunch under different conditions, including in silence, or listening to a story. The women ate more food – on average 300 calories more – while listening to the story compared with eating in silence.

Don't ban your favourite foods
The moment you tell yourself you can't have something – whether it's chocolate, crisps, cake – you want it. Even if

you eat other things you'll still want that forbidden treat and eventually you'll give in and have it anyway. Including your favourite foods in moderation will make your weight-loss plan easier to stick to, if not pleasurable. If you know that you can eat a little of your favourite indulgence every day, you'll stop thinking of it as a forbidden food and then won't want to binge on it. So go ahead and include chocolate or ice cream, but make sure it's only a little.

Simplify your food choices
Research at Tufts University in Massachusetts shows that when people are presented with a wider variety of foods they eat considerably more. Also, when you eat a single food, your eating slows down, you are satiated more quickly and so you eat less. The pleasure of eating a food increases up to the third or fourth bite, and then drops off. If you have lots of different foods on your plate you prolong the sensory pleasure, which stops you feeling full. The message here is to simplify your diet. Place fewer types of foods on your plate. When shopping, stick to your list and ignore the lure of new varieties of ready-made meals and snacks on the shelves.

Curb evening nibbling
Skipping breakfast or lunch (or eating only small amounts) may seem an easy way of saving calories, but not meeting your energy needs during the day and then back-loading at night is the perfect scenario for gaining fat. Levels of hunger hormones rise through the day, leading to an overwhelming desire for food in the evening. Aim to eat two thirds of a day's total calories before your evening meal.

Fill up with soup
Starting your meal with a bowl of soup can cut your calories by 20 per cent compared with eating the main course alone, according to Pennsylvania State University studies. It doesn't matter whether you choose a chunky or a smooth/puréed soup, but it should be a low-calorie variety providing

no more than 150 calories per portion (such as vegetable soup, which was tested in the studies) rather than a creamy one. The fibre and liquid fills your stomach, so you then go on to eat less food.

Start with salad or fruit

Eating a large portion of foods with a low calorie density (such as salad or fresh fruit) as a starter can cut the number of calories you eat in your main meal by 12 per cent, according to a 2004 study at Pennsylvania State University. All that fibre and water takes the edge off your appetite so you eat less of the higher-calorie foods. Take care not to add too much dressing.

Beware of juice and smoothies

Both fruit juice and smoothies contain much higher concentrations of (natural) sugar than the fresh fruit they came from and are less satiating.

When you squeeze the fruit you lose the filling power of fibre. Even crushing it to make a smoothie destroys the cell walls, so you don't have to chew the fruit. This means it's easy to over-consume calories before your hunger is satisfied. Down a glass of orange juice and you'll take in about 120 calories, but if you eat an orange instead you'll save 60 calories, get more fibre and feel more satisfied.

Should overweight children lose weight?

With children, the best approach is to make healthy changes to what they eat and encourage regular physical activity. You shouldn't put them on a diet without the advice of a doctor or dietitian in case they miss out on important nutrients. Overly restricting their food intake often results in them eating high-calorie snacks in secret. Here's how you can help children reach a healthy weight:

Build self-esteem: If you can help children feel more positive about themselves they are more likely to make healthier food choices.

Set a good example: Children are more likely to copy what you do than what you say. Share mealtimes as often as possible and eat the same meals. A 2005 Australian study found that children who ate regular meals with their family were far less likely to be overweight by the age of fourteen. They were also less likely to eat unhealthy snacks and more likely to eat well when they were not at home.

Don't pass your weight worries to your kids: Mothers who worry about their own weight may unknowingly pass an unhealthy attitude towards food to their children. According to a study at Glasgow University involving 100 young children, dieting parents or those who are overanxious about food, may be to blame for their children's unhealthy attitude towards eating and their bodies.

Don't ban any foods: Banning a food only increases children's desire for it and makes it more likely that they will eat it in secret. Allow all foods but explain that certain ones should be eaten only infrequently or kept as occasional treats.

Provide healthy snacks: Don't have biscuits, crisps and chocolate in the house. Make sure there are plenty of healthier alternatives to hand: fresh fruit, low-fat yoghurt, nuts, wholemeal toast and whole-grain breakfast cereals.

Get them moving: Look for ways to incorporate activity into everything they do, and make this as much fun as possible. Walk or cycle with them to and from school. Try to increase the amount of exercise you do together as a family – swimming, playing football, a family walk or bike ride.

Limit time spent watching television: Plan and agree exactly what your children will watch on television and agree on a defined time period. Once the programmes have finished, switch off the television, no matter how much they protest. Don't place a television in your children's bedrooms.

How much is too much TV?

Researchers have shown that children burn fewer calories watching television than if they were reading or drawing a picture! Over 80 per cent watch more than one hour of television each day during the school week, but watching TV for an extra two hours a day increases the chances of obesity by 25 per cent. An American study of six- to eleven-year-olds found that those who watched more than five hours of TV a day were more than four times as likely to be overweight as those who watched two hours or less a day.

Chapter 3

Eat Yourself Fit

I have somehow managed to run three marathons, two in London and one in New York; as well as five 26-mile moonwalks in aid of breast cancer charities. The only way I was able to last the distance was a combination of training and eating properly.

I always made sure I ate a really good breakfast, usually porridge which I ate with semi-skimmed milk, or with the addition of fruit, honey or yoghurt.

Trying to boost your fitness levels with a healthy diet? Knowing what to eat, how much and when is crucial for getting the most out of your fitness regime. Get it right and you'll perform better – and feel terrific. Bad eating habits, on the other hand, will undermine your efforts and set you up for fitness failure.

Planning what you eat before and after exercise is important. A healthy diet will increase your energy and endurance, reduce fatigue and maximise your fitness gains. After exercise, you need to give your body enough of the nutrients it needs for repair and recovery.

I exercise regularly – what are the changes I need to make to my diet?

The main difference between the diet of a regular exerciser and that of a couch potato is the amount of carbohydrate and protein it contains. Carbohydrate, in the form of muscle glycogen, is the main fuel used for virtually all types of exercise. The harder and the more often you exercise the more carbohydrate you'll need. Experts recommend an intake of 5–7g per kg of body weight for active people (exercising 1–2 hours a day). So, for example, a person weighing 60kg would need 300–420g carbohydrate daily. That's equivalent to four slices of bread, a jacket potato, two apples, a generous portion of pasta, a yoghurt and a cereal bar. Not bad, eh!

Should I cut out fats?

Definitely not. Certain fats – the omega-3 fatty acids – are positively beneficial for your performance. They enhance oxygen delivery around your body and even help your body burn fat more efficiently (see page 37, 'Omega-3s'). Aim to have a weekly portion of oily fish (such as salmon or mackerel) or a daily tablespoon of an omega-3-rich oil (flaxseed, rapeseed or a branded omega-3-rich oil).

Should I eat more protein?

If you're exercising seriously three or more times a week, you will need a little extra protein to help repair and build new muscle tissue. Aim to get 1.4 to 1.8g/kg body weight per day if you work out with weights (which translates as between 84 and 108g of protein daily if you weigh 60kg). If you do mainly aerobic activities, 1.2 to 1.4g/kg body weight per day will cover your needs (that's 72 to 84g protein daily if you weigh 60kg). Include two portions of high-protein foods a day, such as meat, poultry, fish, dairy foods, eggs, beans, lentils, grains, nuts, seeds, soya or Quorn. Protein supplements are unnecessary for most exercisers – only serious athletes working out more than three times a week may benefit from the extra protein.

Will extra protein make me stronger?

It's tempting to think that a high-protein diet will make you stronger but the truth is only a resistance training programme together with a balanced diet can make your muscles stronger. Regular exercisers need around 72 to 84g compared with 45g for a non-active person weighing 60kg. Most people get more than the daily requirement for protein from their meals. Two or three portions (each the size of a deck of cards) of lean meat, fish, poultry, beans, lentils, dairy products or Quorn daily will meet your needs. Serious bodybuilders (who need up to 1.8g of protein per kilo of body weight daily) and vegans (who exclude dairy and meat) may need protein drinks or bars to help make up a shortfall in their diet.

Do I need extra vitamins?

Regular exercise increases your vitamin and mineral requirements above the RDAs set for the general population (see page 44, 'Should I take extra vitamins and minerals?'), so you'll need to step up your intake of fresh fruit and vegetables. You'll need extra B-vitamins (found in whole grains, nuts, beans, lentils and lean meat) for energy production. As exercise produces extra free radicals, you'll need more antioxidant nutrients, such as vitamin C and E, too.

When is the best time to eat before exercising?

Ideally, you should have your pre-workout meal two to four hours beforehand. You should feel comfortable – not full and not hungry. According to a study at the University of North

Carolina, eating a moderately high-carbohydrate, low-fat meal three hours before exercise allows you to exercise longer and perform better during a thirty-minute workout than eating six hours beforehand. If you haven't eaten since lunchtime and plan to workout at five or six o'clock, have a light snack fifteen to thirty minutes before training.

What are the best foods to eat before exercise?

Slow burning – or low glycaemic – foods that produce a gradual rise in blood-sugar levels are your best bet before working out. Researchers at the University of Sydney found that cyclists were able to exercise twenty minutes longer after a low-glycaemic meal compared with a high-glycaemic meal. The slower release of energy helped maintain their blood-sugar levels and spare muscle glycogen (stored carbohydrate). Porridge, cereal with milk, a chicken or cheese sandwich, a jacket potato with beans, or pasta with tuna are suitable pre-workout meals.

✳ How to burn more fat

Eating a low GI meal may also help you burn more fat during exercise, according to a 2005 study at Loughborough University. Runners who ate a low GI meal three hours before exercise burned more fat than those who ate a high GI meal with the same amount of carbs. Try fruit and yoghurt, Weetabix with milk, or a baked potato with cheese.

Should I have a pre-workout drink?

If you plan to exercise for longer than an hour, a pre-workout drink or snack rich in carbohydrate, consumed thirty to sixty minutes before exercise, will benefit your performance. Try an apple, a few dried apricots, a handful of sultanas, a smoothie, a pot of yoghurt, 300ml of diluted fruit juice (50/50) or even half a bar (25g) of chocolate. Those extra carbohydrates will help boost your stamina and postpone fatigue.

But for shorter workouts, a pre-exercise snack may not give you any extra benefit. Most of the energy needed for exercise is provided by whatever you have eaten several hours, indeed days, before. A balanced diet that includes enough carbohydrate will produce high levels of glycogen (stored carbohydrate) in your muscles.

Will eating a few sweets before exercise give me a quick energy fix?

Provided you stick to a small portion size, eating sweets (or other high-sugar foods) just before exercise may help maintain blood-sugar levels while you exercise. Although they have a high glycaemic index (GI), a small portion actually gives you a low to moderate glycaemic load (GL) (see page 16, 'What's the difference between the GI and glycaemic load (GL) diets?'). For example, 30g of jelly beans (25g sugar) has a GL of 19 and produces a modest blood-sugar rise, despite its high GI (76). But a 60g portion (or 50g sugar) has a GL of 38 – enough to send your blood-sugar levels soaring. Eating too much sugar just before exercise increases the risk of hypoglycaemia (low blood sugar), faintness and dizziness. So, if you need a pre-exercise boost, stick to small portions of sugary foods before exercise or – better still – opt for lower GI choices such as bananas, grapes or yoghurt drinks.

Does exercising on an empty stomach burn more fat?

If fat loss is your goal, then exercising on an empty stomach – when blood sugar and insulin levels are low – encourages the muscles to burn more calories from fat than carbohydrate. You won't burn more calories but more of the calories you do burn will come from fat. But, according to University of Connecticut researchers, the downside of exercising on an empty stomach is that you will tire sooner and/or exercise at a lower intensity. The result is you burn fewer calories. So if you want to get fitter faster, you will be better off eating a light snack two to four hours before exercise. The resulting rise in blood-glucose levels slows the rate of glycogen depletion, enabling you to exercise harder and longer, and burn more calories. The more calories you burn, the more fat you lose.

I like to run first thing in the morning. Should I force myself to eat?

Many people claim they can't run with food in their stomachs and complain of stitch, nausea or stomach discomfort. It's an individual thing but it is possible to 'train' yourself to run with a small amount of food inside you. The potential benefits are more energy and greater endurance, so try different high-carb options to find what works for you.

Try a slice of toast, a banana, a small cereal or energy bar, a pot of yoghurt or a handful of dried fruit (such as raisins, apricots or sultanas). If you can't face solid food, try a liquid meal: fruit juice (diluted half-and-half with water), a smoothie, flavoured milk or a commercial carbohydrate and protein shake.

In any case, drink a cupful (150–250ml) of water or diluted juice before setting out. This will help rehydrate you after your night's fast and reduce the risk of dehydration during your workout.

If you cannot eat anything at all, make sure you eat plenty the day before and for breakfast after your workout.

✴ Pre-exercise snacks

- Fresh fruit
- Wholemeal toast with honey
- Cereal bar
- Fruit yoghurt
- Dried fruit
- Cereal with milk

Pre-exercise meals

Eat two to four hours before exercise:

- Sandwich/roll/bagel/wrap filled with chicken, fish, cheese, egg or peanut butter
- Jacket potato with beans, cheese, tuna, coleslaw or chicken
- Pasta with tomato-based pasta sauce, vegetables and cheese
- Macaroni cheese with salad
- Rice with chicken or fish and vegetables
- Porridge made with milk
- Whole-grain cereal with milk or yoghurt

Should you eat anything during exercise?

Only if you are exercising for more than ninety minutes. Having an extra 30 to 60g of carbohydrate per hour while exercising helps maintain your blood-glucose level, delay fatigue and increase your endurance, according to studies at the University of Texas. Start refuelling after about thirty minutes and continue at regular intervals. Choose high GI carbohydrates, which convert into blood sugar rapidly. Sports drinks, energy gels and energy bars are popular with athletes, but bananas, fruit bars, cereal or breakfast bars, low-fat biscuits (e.g. fig rolls), malt loaf, dried fruit and chocolate work equally well.

How much should I drink during exercise?

According to studies with athletes at the University of Aberdeen, if you can replace at least 80 per cent of your fluid loss or keep within 1 per cent of your body weight, then your performance won't be affected. Exactly how much you need to drink depends on how heavily you are sweating. Most people lose around 750 to 1,000ml per hour so you'll need to put back around 600 to 800ml in that time. However, the old mantra to drink as much as possible during exercise has been replaced with the advice to listen to your body and drink when you feel thirsty (see below 'Is it possible to over-hydrate during exercise?').

Is it possible to over-hydrate during exercise?

Yes. Following a (very small) number of cases of hyponatraemia (a dangerous condition caused by drinking too much water) during the London marathon, sports medicine experts now caution against over-hydrating yourself in events lasting longer than four hours. Constantly drinking water may dilute your blood so that your sodium levels fall. Although it is quite rare it is potentially fatal. The American College of Sports Medicine (ACSM) and USA Track & Field advise drinking when you're thirsty or drinking only to the point at which you're maintaining your weight, not gaining weight. Sports drinks are better than water if you're running a marathon because their sodium content will prevent hyponatraemia.

✳ What to consume during prolonged exercise

- O Isotonic sports drink
- O Energy bar*

O Diluted fruit juice (50/50 juice and water)
O Banana*
O Raisins*
O Sports gel*
* Plus water

What are the best foods to eat after exercising?

Kick-start your recovery with a high-carbohydrate, high GI snack or drink within two hours of exercise. Your muscles replenish their glycogen stores one and a half times faster during this two-hour window so virtually all the carbohydrates you eat during this time will go straight to your muscle cells, not to your fat cells, according to research from Texas University. The Texas researchers recommend eating around 1g for each 1kg of your body weight – that's 60g if you weigh 60kg, equivalent to a jam sandwich (two slices of bread with a tablespoon of jam) or two and a half slices of malt loaf.

✳ Best snacks after exercise

O Isotonic sports drink
O Fruit smoothie or low-fat milkshake
O Baked potato with cottage cheese or tuna
O Tuna, chicken or cheese sandwich
O Breakfast cereal with low-fat milk
O Dried fruit and nuts
O Fresh fruit and a fruit yoghurt
O Cereal bar
O Yoghurt drink

How much should I drink after exercising?

After working out, the ADA/ACSM recommend drinking at least 450 to 675ml for every 0.5kg of body weight lost during exercise. Monitor your urine. Drink plenty of fluids until your urine is pale yellow. Aim for about 250ml of fluid immediately after exercise, and then continue drinking at regular intervals.

Water is the best sports drink if you are exercising for less than one hour. But for longer sessions, an isotonic sports drink containing 4 to 8g/100ml will help maintain blood-sugar levels, and combat fatigue. Make your own isotonic drink by diluting fruit juice with one or two parts of water.

I get starving after a workout – how can I avoid binge eating?

Your increased appetite is your body's way of telling you to eat. After a hard workout, you need to replace the fuel you have just used – but no more than that! Combining protein with carbohydrate in your post-workout snack or meal not only speeds glycogen recovery and muscle repair compared with eating carbohydrate alone, but also helps to blunt your appetite. Protein is the most effective nutrient for switching off hunger signals so it helps to stop you overeating. Try a meal-replacement shake (protein and carbohydrate shake), home-made milkshake, a pot of yoghurt, a cottage cheese sandwich, or a handful of dried fruit and nuts.

Is it true that calories I eat after a workout won't be stored as fat?

Not exactly. Carbohydrate eaten after exercise is preferentially stored as glycogen but only if your intake matches the glycogen storage rate. The enzymes in your muscles turn carbohydrates into glycogen but can only process around 50 to 70g per two hours after exercise. Eating more than this risks fat storage as the resulting carbohydrate 'overspill' will be converted into fat. But it's not just how much you eat that matters, you also have to consider the GI of your post-exercise meal. High GI carbohydrates – sugar, biscuits, white bread or rice cakes – provoke a rapid release of insulin, which forces carbohydrates into your fat cells as well as glycogen cells. The key to minimising fat storage after a workout is to eat low GI meals – a balance of carbohydrate, protein and healthy fat – such as jacket potatoes, fish and salad with a little olive oil.

Should I eat anything after exercise if it's late in the evening?

Yes. Whether you exercise early in the day or late in the evening, you need to refuel your muscles. Skipping that post-workout meal will delay your recovery and leave you feeling sluggish the next day. Provided you don't overeat, these calories will not be turned into fat. After working out, have a drink (water, diluted juice or a sports drink) straight away and then have a snack or light meal. Try a smoothie, a milkshake, toast with peanut butter, or a jacket potato with tuna. Remember to count this snack towards your total daily calories, so you won't gain weight, and plan ahead to ensure you have all the right foods and ingredients to hand.

Do I need supplements?

If you exercise several times a week, your requirements for many vitamins and minerals will be greater than the RDAs, so a multivitamin supplement may help top up any shortfall in your diet. But don't believe the hype of other sports supplements – some can actually be harmful. 'Fat-burners', for example, may contain substances that have undesirable side effects such as tachycardia, nausea, diarrhoea and headaches, and will invariably adversely affect your exercise performance. A 2001 International

Olympic Committee-funded survey of 634 supplements found 15 per cent were contaminated with banned substances, including steroids. UK Sport and the British Olympic Association strictly advise athletes against taking *any* supplements.

I sweat heavily during exercise – should I have extra salt?

It's unlikely that your salt needs are higher than normal. Salt losses in sweat are relatively small, even when exercising in very hot weather. People in some countries survive on a fraction of the amount of salt eaten by people in the UK. So there's no need to eat extra salt – it's more important to drink plenty of water to keep your body hydrated. The muscle cramps that sometimes follow exercise are due to dehydration, not lack of salt. To prevent cramps, drink plenty of water on hot days and before, during and after exercise. This will also help to even out the water–sodium ratio in the body.

Can my body adapt to dehydration during exercise?

It's a myth that you can 'train' yourself to exercise without drinking much. The body doesn't adapt to dehydration. You increase the risk of health problems and should not ignore the warning signs (see box 'Warning signs of dehydration'). Losing the equivalent of 2 per cent of your body weight as sweat – that's 1.4kg loss if you weigh 70kg – results in a 10 to 20 per cent drop in your performance. When you become dehydrated, exercise feels harder, endurance is reduced and you will tire sooner. In severe cases, it can result in vomiting and heat exhaustion. Prevent dehydration by drinking before and during exercise.

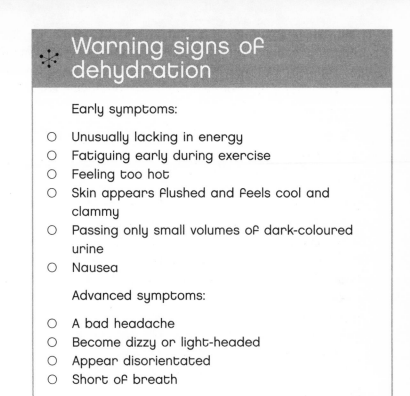

Warning signs of dehydration

Early symptoms:

- ○ Unusually lacking in energy
- ○ Fatiguing early during exercise
- ○ Feeling too hot
- ○ Skin appears flushed and feels cool and clammy
- ○ Passing only small volumes of dark-coloured urine
- ○ Nausea

Advanced symptoms:

- ○ A bad headache
- ○ Become dizzy or light-headed
- ○ Appear disorientated
- ○ Short of breath

What should I do if I get dehydrated?

Stop exercising. If you are experiencing early symptoms of dehydration (see box 'Warning signs of dehydration'), drink 100–200ml water or sports drink every 10–15 minutes. But if you have more advanced symptoms, you should also seek professional help.

Do sports drinks work?

Sports drinks may help improve your endurance during activities lasting longer than sixty minutes. Research from the University of Texas found that drinking water during one hour of cycling improved performance by 6 per cent compared with no water, but drinking a sports drink resulted in a 12 per cent improvement on performance. Researchers at the University of Loughborough found that when runners drank a sports drink (containing 5.5g carbohydrate per 100ml), they improved their running time by nearly four minutes over 42km compared with drinking water.

What's special about sports drinks then?

They are basically a concoction of sugar, water and sodium (these are the 'active' ingredients) designed to speed fluid uptake and fuel your muscles. The optimal concentration of sugars is believed to be around 40 to 80g per litre (although lower concentrations will also help the water get into your system faster than plain water). The sodium increases the urge to drink and improves the drink's taste (whereas plain water quenches your thirst before you're fully rehydrated). It also helps the body hold on to more water during and after exercise. The ideal concentration is around 0.5 to 0.7g of sodium per litre.

However, other minerals and vitamins found in certain sports drinks have no immediate effect on your performance – they simply add to your overall daily intake. On the downside, many brands contain artificial sweeteners, preservatives and colours, which, although considered safe by the FSA, may cause adverse reactions in a few people. The long-term risks of artificial additives are unknown.

Try making your own isotonic sports drink by mixing 500ml of fruit juice with 500ml of water. If you plan to exercise hard for longer than one hour and sweat losses are likely to be high, add 1.0 to 1.5g (one eighth to one quarter of a teaspoon) of salt. But count this salt towards your daily 6g maximum.

Can energy gels help me exercise longer?

Energy gels – squeezy sachets of concentrated sugar and maltodextrin – provide a convenient way of consuming carbohydrate on the run. But they only benefit your performance during endurance exercise lasting longer than an hour. Studies show that consuming 30 to 60g of carbohydrate per hour during prolonged exercise delays fatigue and improves endurance. This translates into one or two sachets per hour. One study showed that gels have a similar effect on blood-sugar levels and performance as sports drinks. But you need to drink around 350ml of water with each 25g of gel – this effectively dilutes it down to a 7 per cent sugar solution in your stomach. Try half a gel with 175ml (six big gulps) every fifteen to thirty minutes. On the downside, some people dislike their texture, sweetness and intensity of flavour.

Would energy drinks give me more energy?

Only in the sense that energy equals calories. The term energy refers to the high energy or calorie content of the drink. Energy drinks typically contain higher concentrations of carbohydrate (sugars and maltodextrin) than ordinary sports drinks, usually between 8 and 20g per 100ml. They are designed to help maintain blood-glucose levels, replenish fluid losses and delay fatigue during long periods of intense exercise. So you may benefit from an energy drink if you exercise hard for more than sixty minutes. But there's little point in having an energy drink if you exercise for less than this.

Some energy drinks also contain caffeine to help increase endurance. Caffeine steps up adrenaline release, which raises blood levels of fatty acids, thus sparing muscle glycogen and delaying fatigue.

Aim to drink 300 to 450ml per hour – sip around 100ml every 15 minutes.

I train with weights – will protein supplements help me build muscle?

Protein supplements, whether in the form of drinks or bars, are essentially a concentrated source of protein, based on milk-derived protein (such as whey and casein), and designed to supplement your usual food intake. Most regular exercisers can get enough protein from two to four daily portions of meat, chicken, fish, dairy products, eggs and pulses. Protein supplements would only benefit you if you have particularly high protein requirements (e.g. you do strength training), and/or you cannot consume enough protein from food alone. Estimate your daily protein intake from food and compare that with your protein requirement. Experts recommend an intake between 1.2 and 1.4g/kg of body weight per day for endurance athletes, and 1.4 and 1.8g/kg of body weight per day for strength athletes. For example, a strength athlete weighing 80kg may need as much as 144g protein a day. This may be difficult to get from food alone. Only if there is a consistent protein shortfall should you consider adding supplements.

How should I prepare for a competition?

What you eat and drink during the week before a competition can make a big difference to your performance, particularly for endurance events and competitions lasting more than ninety minutes. The idea with a pre-competition eating strategy is to maximise your muscle glycogen stores and keep yourself well hydrated. Here's how to do it:

The week before

Train less – Taper your training over the last few days of the week and, ideally, rest completely for the last day or two. This allows full recovery of your muscle glycogen stores.

Carb up – Increase the amount of carbohydrate in your diet and reduce the fat calories by a corresponding amount. This helps boost your glycogen levels and gives you more fuel for the event.

Drink plenty – Make sure you drink at least two litres per day. Dehydration is cumulative, so if you fail to drink enough over a few days, the effects carry over, which means you could be dehydrated on the day of the event.

The day before

Eat little and often – Small frequent meals are easier to digest and prevent you feeling 'heavy' or 'bloated' on the day of the competition. Avoid big meals and don't eat too much of any food.

Don't try any new foods – The last thing you want before a race is a stomach upset, so play it safe by sticking to familiar foods. Choose fairly plain foods and avoid spicy and salty foods.

Keep drinking – Drink plenty of fluids throughout the day. Your urine should be pale or almost clear.

Avoid gas! – Steer clear of gas-forming foods, such as baked beans, lentils and other pulses, cauliflower, Brussels sprouts, bran cereals and spicy foods. Eating them could give you an uncomfortable time the next day!

Don't party – Do not overindulge the evening before your race. A large meal – even if it's high in carbohydrate – could make you feel sluggish the next day. If you must drink alcohol, restrict yourself to a maximum of one or two units, otherwise you risk dehydration and a hangover on race day. Better still, avoid alcohol altogether.

On race day

Eat a healthy breakfast – Eat your pre-race meal two to four hours before the start of your race. Skipping that pre-race meal may leave you low in energy.

Pre-race meals

- ○ Cereal with dried fruit and milk
- ○ Scrambled egg on toast
- ○ Porridge with fruit
- ○ Toasted bagels or muffins and milky drink
- ○ Smoothie made with fruit and yoghurt

Go easy on the fibre! – Steer clear of bran and high-fibre cereals, especially if you are feeling nervous. Cereal fibre may loosen the stools and cause more bowel movements than normal.

Drink – Make sure you are fully hydrated by drinking plenty of water before the competition. Your urine should be a very pale yellow colour.

During the competition
If you'll be competing for longer than thirty minutes, you'll need to drink; longer than ninety minutes and you'll also need extra carbohydrate.

Drink – Aim to drink little and often, aiming for 150 to 350ml every 15 to 20 minutes during endurance events; or according to your thirst.

Drink whatever you used in training – As a rule of thumb, water is fine for events lasting sixty to ninety minutes; sports drinks are better for longer events. But do not try anything different – even it's freely provided – in case it doesn't agree with you under race conditions.

Fuel up – For events longer than ninety minutes you will need extra carbohydrate – try sports drinks, energy drinks, energy gels, bars or dried fruit with plenty of water. But experiment in training first.

✳ Post-race snacks

- ○ Smoothie or milkshake
- ○ Yoghurt drink
- ○ Fresh fruit
- ○ Dried fruit and nuts
- ○ Honey or jam sandwich

How can I avoid 'hitting the wall' during a marathon?

'Hitting the wall' occurs when you have used up all the glycogen in your muscles and liver and your blood-sugar level plummets. In other words, you have used up all your energy. You may feel weak, dizzy, nauseous and disorientated. To avoid this, have extra carbohydrate at regular intervals during the race, aiming for 30 to 60g per hour. That's equivalent to drinking 500 to 1,000ml of sports drink (containing 60g carbohydrate/litre), one or two energy bars, two or three bananas, or a couple of energy gels. This should help to keep your blood-sugar levels steady and fuel your muscles during that last stage of the race.

I have no appetite after a run and certainly don't feel like eating. Should I wait until I'm hungry or force myself to eat?

A lot of runners find they have little appetite after racing. Running (along with other types of intense exercise) elevates your temperature and diverts blood away from your digestive system, which in turn depresses your appetite. If you want to recover faster, you should consume some carbohydrate within the first thirty minutes after a race or, at the very least, within two hours. Try a liquid meal, such as a meal-replacement shake, milkshake, smoothie or yoghurt drink. You'll feel better for it the next day.

How much exercise should children get?

It's important for kids to move for at least one hour every day. It doesn't have to be done in one go – they can do four fifteen-minute periods of activity, three twenty-minutes or two thirty-minutes. This could include walking to and from school, playing with their friends, playing sport or unstructured play such as ball games, 'chase' and hide and seek, or sports activities. Older children aged eleven to sixteen years should also aim to do three sessions per week of continuous vigorous activity lasting at least twenty minutes, e.g. jogging, swimming, cycling, dancing or football.

What's the best way for kids to exercise?

Get kids active at every opportunity. Try and build activity into their daily routine: walking to and from school and other nearby places, riding a bike to visit friends and playing active games will help them see exercise as a way of life. Lead by example and show your child that you value activity by taking part yourself. There is nothing more guaranteed to get children interested in a sport than seeing Mum and Dad enjoying it. Keep it fun – it is vital they have fun with any activities they do. If they are enthusiastic about activity or sport they'll stick to it. Provide plenty of play equipment at home – hoppers, balls, basketball or netball rings, scooters, bikes and skipping ropes.

Have a think about getting them to:

○ Walk or cycle to school.
○ Try activities such as swimming, playing football, Frisbee, tennis, a family bike ride or walk.
○ Add purpose to activities – walking the dog, joining a swimming club or entering family charity sports events.
○ Help with household chores (like vacuuming and washing the car) and gardening.
○ Enjoy a wide range of sports — football, racket games, gymnastics, dance lessons and swimming are all suitable for under-elevens; for older children, athletics, roller-skating, hockey, tennis, badminton, netball, jogging and sailing are also suitable.
○ Practise skills such as running, jumping, throwing, catching and kicking, either with you or with friends.
○ Join active clubs at school – football, netball or tennis (ask your children's teacher what is on offer), or after-school

activity sports clubs, activities at the leisure centre, at local community centres or local sports clubs.

✳ Five top action tips

- Give them plenty of support and encouragement – but don't allow your children's sport to become your obsession.
- It is important children learn a good range of movement skills – running, throwing, catching – and not just skills that are specific to one sport.
- The focus, especially with the under-twelves, should be on enjoyment.
- Children under twelve should try a range of sports and not begin to specialise until they are at least eleven.
- If training for a sport is started too early, children can burn out either physically (through injury or fatigue) or mentally (through boredom or stress) by their teens.

Chapter 4

The Power of Food

We all know that our mood affects what we eat. If I am feeling stressed, I have a tendency to head straight for the biscuit tin, so I try and make sure there are plenty of bananas, berries and chopped carrot to hand to munch on instead. And I always crave chocolate, sweets and also really salty stuff when I am pre-menstrual – eating these foods can bring instant satisfaction, but it's always followed by a hellish crash which leaves me feeling exhausted, so I try and have healthy alternatives.

But the link between food and mood goes much further than this, and what we eat can have a powerful effect on how we feel; it can lift our mood, making us feel good, or it can have the opposite effect, depressing our mood. It can make us feel calm, sleepy or irritable. It can ease the symptoms of pre-menstrual syndrome. It can also help combat problems such as low energy levels, fatigue, insomnia, migraines and infertility; boost our brain power and memory; improve alertness and concentration; boost our immunity; and even prevent wrinkles, so there's no need to spend vast amounts of money on the latest anti-ageing product!

Amid all the food scares and conflicting claims, this chapter explains why it's a good idea to eat more of some foods . . . and less of others.

Diet and mood

Can eating certain foods really alter your mood?

The answer is yes – but obviously not in the same way as alcohol or drugs! Scientists have shown that what you eat (or don't eat) may lift or depress your mood, cause fatigue or even exacerbate depression. According to studies at the Rochester Institute of Technology in New York, certain nutrients in foods are precursors to brain chemical messengers (neurotransmitters) – serotonin and dopamine – which can alter levels of alertness, pain perception and anxiety. Serotonin reduces pain, produces a sense of calm and, at high levels, induces sleep. Dopamine increases levels of alertness and energy.

What can I eat to make me feel alert?

To boost alertness, include a little extra protein in your meal. High-protein foods such as fish, poultry, meat, dairy products and eggs contain the amino acid tyrosine. This ups the body's production of dopamine, which in turn increases levels of alertness and energy.

Caffeine, found in coffee, tea, cola and certain energy drinks, acts as a stimulant and can also increase concentration and alertness. People who drink a coffee with breakfast perform better during the morning and tend to be more upbeat, according to researchers. But drinking more than three cups a day can make you feel more stressed.

What can I eat to make me feel calm?

Eat more carbs. These trigger the production of insulin, which lowers levels of all amino acids in the bloodstream except tryptophan. This amino acid is normally crowded out by other amino acids competing to cross the blood–brain barrier. But when the other amino acids are out of the way, it enters the brain where it is converted into mood-boosting serotonin. So, for instant calm, opt for a banana, a dish of plain pasta, rice, potatoes or cereal. But go easy on portion sizes at lunch if you want to stay alert. Eating too much carbohydrate can induce sleepiness and cause a post-lunch dip in energy.

Could my diet be making me feel irritable – and how can I avoid this?

When blood-sugar levels start to dip, you're more likely to experience a change in your mood and feel irritable. You can avoid this by choosing foods that release their energy slowly. These foods have a low glycaemic index (see page 14 for an explanation of glycaemic index) and include porridge, beans, most fruits, pasta and vegetables. A study at the University of Cardiff found that eating a wholemeal breakfast cereal for breakfast each day helped people feel less stressed and generally happier than those who had a 'normal' breakfast. High GI foods, which are best avoided, include white bread, white rice and sugary drinks. Dividing your daily food intake into several smaller meals will also help maintain steady levels of blood sugar – and a good mood.

Is there anything I can eat to help pick me up when I'm feeling low?

Oily fish such as salmon, sardines, pilchards and mackerel contain omega-3 oils, have been shown to help counter anxiety and generally improve wellbeing. In research carried out in Israel, omega-3 oils were found to be more effective in reducing symptoms of depression than antidepressant medication. They may also stave off dementia, help memory and alertness, as well as being beneficial for the circulation. Non-fish sources of omega-3s include walnuts, soya, rapeseed oil and omega-3 eggs.

Is there any link between diet and depression?

Studies have suggested that not having enough of the vitamin folic acid can increase the chances of depression, low moods and fatigue. Low levels of folic acid cause serotonin levels in the brain to drop. Patients with depression are much more likely to have folic acid deficiency than the rest of the population. Folic acid also protects against Alzheimer's and Parkinson's diseases. Help counter depression by getting the RDA of 200 micrograms daily, equivalent to three servings of fortified breakfast cereal. Other food sources include dark-green leafy vegetables, oranges, wholemeal bread, yeast extract, nuts and pulses.

Minor deficiencies of the B-vitamins thiamin and niacin can also cause depression, irritability and fatigue. Wholemeal bread and cereals, pulses and nuts are good sources of both.

Make sure you get enough selenium too. Low intakes may also increase the chances of depression and a negative mood. Just two Brazil nuts will give you your daily needs for selenium. Other food sources include cereals, vegetables, dairy products, meat and eggs.

Diet and brain power

Can my diet make me brainier?

Eating certain foods may help keep your mind sharp and prevent age-related memory loss. The strongest evidence is for omega-3 fatty acids, which are the primary building blocks of the brain. These oils boost blood flow in the brain, boost your speed of thought and improve memory. Aim to have at least one weekly portion of oily fish, such as salmon, sardines, pilchards, mackerel, herring and kippers. They are the richest source of omega-3s, but other foods include walnuts, olive, rapeseed and flaxseed oil.

Vitamin B12 and folic acid are thought to protect against Alzheimer's and Parkinson's diseases, so make sure you include plenty of spinach and green leafy vegetables in your diet. These foods are the best sources, as well as lean meat, fish, canned beans and lentils, dairy products and grains. Lean meat, poultry, fish, whole grains, canned beans and lentils are rich in B-vitamins, which appear to help control inflammation and may play a role in the development of new brain cells.

Bright-coloured fruits and vegetables, especially blueberries, strawberries, plums, raspberries and blackcurrant (fresh, canned or frozen), are high in antioxidants. Research suggests they may improve short-term memory.

A good mix of fruit and veg helps keep the brain well oxygenated and improves mental alertness, thanks to their high content of potassium and vitamin C.

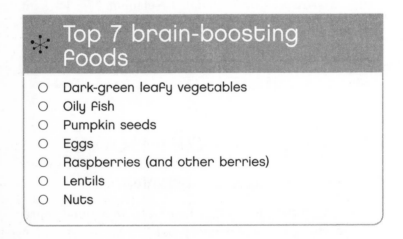

Top 7 brain-boosting foods

- O Dark-green leafy vegetables
- O Oily fish
- O Pumpkin seeds
- O Eggs
- O Raspberries (and other berries)
- O Lentils
- O Nuts

Are there any foods to help boost my memory?

Including eggs in your diet may help boost your memory and concentration. They are a rich source of choline. Studies have shown that college students who were given 3–4g of choline one hour before taking memory tests scored higher than those who hadn't taken any. Choline is an amino acid that your body converts into the brain neurotransmitter acetylcholine, which is linked to memory. Low levels of acetylcholine may impair memory and are associated with Alzheimer's disease.

Diet and insomnia

What can I eat for a better night's sleep?

Certain foods may help you get a more restful night's sleep; others may keep you awake. Good sleep-promoting foods are those that contain high levels of tryptophan: milk, yoghurt, cheese, fish, poultry, meat, lentils, beans, nuts and seeds. This amino acid helps your body produce serotonin, which makes you feel sleepy.

For a bigger serotonin boost, eat a tryptophan-rich food along with a carbohydrate-rich food, such as a meal of egg on toast. The carbohydrates allow your body to process the tryptophan more easily and, therefore, make more serotonin. But a high-protein meal with no carbohydrates may keep you awake, since protein-rich foods also contain tyrosine, which boosts alertness (see page 137, 'Diet and mood'). So, for restful sleep, opt for a meal containing both protein (tryptophan) and carbohydrates in the evening. Adding calcium (found in milk, yoghurt and cheese) will help further. Calcium helps your brain use tryptophan to make melatonin, another sleep-inducing brain chemical. That's why a milky drink – which contains both tryptophan and calcium – is one of the best sleep-inducing foods.

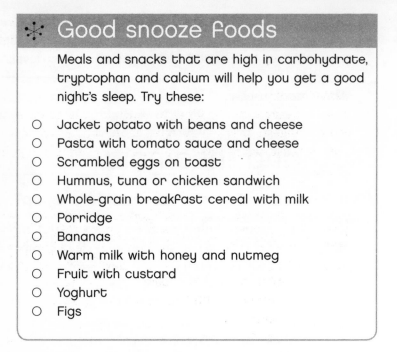

Good snooze foods

Meals and snacks that are high in carbohydrate, tryptophan and calcium will help you get a good night's sleep. Try these:

- Jacket potato with beans and cheese
- Pasta with tomato sauce and cheese
- Scrambled eggs on toast
- Hummus, tuna or chicken sandwich
- Whole-grain breakfast cereal with milk
- Porridge
- Bananas
- Warm milk with honey and nutmeg
- Fruit with custard
- Yoghurt
- Figs

Which foods should I avoid before bed?

Some foods and drinks can keep you awake at night or cause disrupted sleep. Here are the main culprits to avoid:

Caffeine-containing drinks

Drinking coffee, tea, cola or any other caffeine-containing drink in the evening is likely to make it difficult to sleep well. Caffeine is a stimulant, which speeds up the action of the nervous system, ups the heart rate and breathing rate – the opposite of what you want to happen before you go to sleep. Since it takes about six hours for the effects of caffeine to wear off, coffee drunk in the morning or around lunchtime probably won't interfere with your sleep.

Alcohol

Avoid alcoholic drinks before bed. A nightcap might help you get to sleep but your peaceful sleep may last only three or four hours. You then tend to wake up when the sedative effects have worn off, and then experience disrupted sleep. The reason for this is that alcohol keeps you in the light stages of sleep but prevents deep sleep.

Heavy meals
Avoid a heavy meal too close to bedtime. A large meal can cause indigestion that interferes with your sleep. Try to leave at least two or three hours between eating and going to bed.

✳ How to get a good night's sleep

- Establish a sleep schedule – go to bed and wake at the same time each day, even at weekends.
- Relax before bed – take time to unwind with a relaxing activity such as reading or listening to music.
- Avoid caffeine or alcohol before bedtime.
- Have a good sleeping environment – get rid of distractions such as noise, bright lights, an uncomfortable bed, a TV or computer in the bedroom. A cooler temperature in the bedroom promotes sleep.
- Don't exercise vigorously too late in the evening – the adrenaline boost may disrupt sleep patterns.
- Avoid large meals before bedtime.
- Don't take late-afternoon naps – it'll make it harder to fall asleep at night.
- Don't lie in bed awake – if you find yourself still awake after twenty minutes, get up and move somewhere else or do a relaxing activity until you feel sleepy.

Is it true that extra sleep helps people lose weight?

Not getting enough sleep increases your risk of becoming overweight. According to a 2004 study at Columbia University, people who slept nine hours or more had, on average, a significantly lower body mass index than those who slept five hours or less. It's to do with two hormones, ghrelin and leptin, that control appetite. A lack of sleep boosts levels of ghrelin (which stimulates your appetite), while lowering levels of leptin (which suppresses appetite). This hormonal imbalance sends a signal to the brain that more food is needed when, in fact, enough has been eaten. Research at the University of Chicago also shows that sleeping for four hours or less increases levels of another hormone, cortisol, which makes you feel hungry in the evening rather than sleepy.

Diet and migraine

I get frequent headaches – could these be triggered by my diet?

Headaches can be caused by many things, including illness, stress and lack of sleep. They may also be triggered by several common foods, and simply changing your diet could be the most effective treatment. Once you and your doctor have ruled out other potentially more serious causes for your headaches, take a look at what you eat every day and see if eliminating common trigger foods eliminates your headaches.

Too much of a certain food or substance contained in a food, can cause symptoms to develop, as can sudden withdrawal from that food or substances. Common substances in food that can bring on headaches include:

○   Monosodium glutamate – a common flavour enhancer

found in Chinese food, soy sauce, pepperoni and packet snack foods. It is also found naturally in Camembert cheese, Parmesan cheese, mushrooms and tomatoes.

○ Nitrites – these preservatives are found in processed meats such as bacon, ham, and pepperoni.

○ Amines – these are found in mature cheese, shellfish, strawberries, red wine, chocolate and spinach.

○ Aspartame – this artificial sweetener, which changes ratios of amino acids in the blood, is found in many drinks and 'diet' foods. It may lower serotonin and trigger headaches

If you suspect a food may be causing your headaches it is best to consult your GP or healthcare professional to ensure a proper diagnosis.

Why do I get a headache if I skip a meal?

If you go for several hours without food, your blood-sugar level can drop too low for your brain to function comfortably. To boost the supply of glucose to the brain, your body releases hormones, which may also cause an increase in blood pressure because they narrow the arteries. This narrowing of the arteries can result in a headache.

Could sugar be causing my headaches?

A rapid rise in blood-sugar levels – caused by consuming lots of high GI foods or drinks – triggers a surge in insulin levels, which sometimes may be followed by a sudden drop in blood sugar. The drop in blood sugar may cause the arteries in the head to constrict, triggering a headache.

Is it true that coffee causes headaches?

Yes, either too much or, ironically, too little caffeine (caffeine withdrawal) may be the cause of headaches in some people. Caffeine, found in coffee, tea, colas and some energy drinks, as well some medications, constricts the diameter of the arteries and this can exacerbate headaches. The body builds up a tolerance to caffeine over time by producing the chemical adenosine, which helps regulate the diameter of the arteries in the head. But when you stop consuming caffeine, the high levels of adenosine will make your arteries dilate. The excessive blood flow may cause a throbbing headache.

✳ How to avoid headaches

- O Eat little and often in order to prevent blood-sugar fluctuations.
- O Avoid high GI foods or at least consume them in smaller amounts, or with a low GI food.
- O Don't stop caffeine suddenly. Gradually reduce over a period of days, weeks or even months.
- O Drink plenty – dehydration can cause headaches.
- O Read food labels carefully to avoid trigger foods.
- O Avoid stress, which is a key headache trigger.
- O Get plenty of sleep – sleep deprivation can cause headaches.

Headache-fighting foods

Some foods may help alleviate headaches. These include:

- O Fish and fish oils – these are anti-inflammatory and may help prevent headaches, so try to eat mackerel, salmon or sardines regularly.
- O Ginger – take as tablets, use it in cooking, or infuse in boiling water and have as tea.
- O Feverfew – available as tablets, or the herb can be infused in boiling water for a pain-relieving tea (pregnant women should avoid feverfew).

Diet and Fertility

Are there any special foods that may help increase my chances of pregnancy?

Eating a healthy diet can greatly increase your chances of getting pregnant. It helps ensure normal levels of hormones in your body and improves the health of your reproductive system. According to scientists at the Harvard School of Public Health, eating certain foods can increase your fertility while others can lead to problems getting pregnant. Make sure your diet contains the following:

Green leafy vegetables – these contain folic acid, important for a healthy reproductive system as well as preventing birth defects such as spina bifida. Other good sources are Brussels sprouts, broccoli and Marmite.

Beans and lentils – their high content of hormone-balancing phyto-oestrogens increases fertility. These foods are also rich in iron as are red meat, egg yolk and dried apricots. Low iron levels are linked to an increased risk of infertility.

Milk, yoghurt, cheese – a 2007 US study found that women who ate two or more portions of full-fat dairy produce such as milk, cheese (or even ice cream) had a 27 per cent lower risk of infertility due to lack of ovulation, compared with women who ate low-fat dairy produce.

Oranges – the high levels of vitamin C found in oranges, as well as peppers, berries and green leafy vegetables, benefit both female and male fertility.

Whole grains (wholemeal bread, oats and whole-grain cereals) – their B-vitamins and iron boost fertility.

Nuts, avocados, oily fish and olive oil – foods that contain monounsaturated and omega-3 fats rather than artery-clogging trans fats, boost your pregnancy chances.

Organic foods – choosing organic foods wherever possible will help avoid xenoestrogens, a type of oestrogen found in environmental chemicals and pesticides that may disrupt the hormonal balance in women and lead to infertility.

What should I avoid eating if I want to get pregnant?

Foods high in saturated and trans fat may hinder your chances of getting pregnant because of their link with obesity. Being overweight reduces fertility. Caffeine has been linked to decreased fertility in both men and women, so limit your intake to no more than two daily cups of coffee – too much caffeine makes it harder for the fertilised egg to grab a hold. Alcohol also reduces your chances of getting pregnant. Drinking more than five units a week reduces fertility by up to 50 per cent, and drinking when pregnant increases the risk of birth defects and low birth weight. Never diet when trying to become pregnant. Being underweight reduces fertility, and can lead to pregnancy complications, miscarriage and delivery problems. Shark, swordfish and merlin should be avoided completely because they contain high levels of mercury, which is toxic to the developing foetus. You should also limit tuna to two weekly portions.

I'm overweight – could this reduce my fertility?

Being overweight or underweight significantly reduces your chances of getting pregnant. A 2007 study at the University of Adelaide looked at weight and its relation to fertility in Australia and found a strong association between overweight and infertility. Overweight women are also more likely to develop polycystic ovary syndrome and, even if women do become pregnant, they are more likely to suffer problems such as pregnancy-related diabetes, miscarriage, birth complications and birth abnormalities.

Similarly, if you are underweight, you also risk infertility. The study at the University of Adelaide found that women who were classified as underweight had a rate of infertility that was significantly higher than women of normal weight. Underweight women tend to have irregular menstrual cycles and irregular ovulation. Often, normal ovulation can be interrupted and menstruation may stop completely. This would obviously prevent conception. The irregularity of the menstrual cycles can affect the lining of the uterus, making it inadequate to support a pregnancy. Even if conception were to occur, the woman would be likely to miscarry the baby. When an eating disorder is present, ovulation can stop for a long period of time, making pregnancy impossible.

I've read that your diet can increase your chances of having a boy or a girl – is this true?

A 2008 study from Exeter University suggested that you can influence the gender of your baby by what you eat. The researchers found that women who consumed the most calories were more likely to have a boy, while those who consumed the fewest calories were more likely to have a girl. However, these findings should not be treated too seriously. If it were true, then in countries with lots of food nearly all the babies should be boys and in poorer countries nearly all should be girls. Whether you have a boy or girl is down to genetics, not what you eat.

Diet and pregnancy

What should I eat during my pregnancy?

Eating a healthy diet will help you cope with the physical challenges of pregnancy and you'll also be catering for a baby who's going to make big demands of you. In addition to the main food groups, you'll need to boost your intake of folic acid. Take a daily 400 microgram folic acid supplement, ideally before conception and then until the twelfth week of your pregnancy, to prevent neural tube defects. You should also eat foods containing folate such as chickpeas, dark-green vegetables, brown rice, lentils and fortified breakfast cereals.

Step up your iron intake – this mineral will support the increase in blood volume. Good sources are red meat (but avoid liver), beans and lentils, wholemeal bread, spinach and other green leafy vegetables. Have a source of vitamin C (fruit or vegetables or fruit juice) with your meal to help your body absorb iron.

Your body needs a little extra protein (6g) each day. Two servings of poultry, lean meat, fish, eggs, beans or lentils should cover it.

But don't 'eat for two'. From six months onwards a modest 200 calories a day is all the extra you need.

What foods should I avoid during pregnancy?

High levels of vitamin A can cause abnormalities in babies, so experts advise avoiding supplements containing vitamin A and fish-liver oil, as well as liver, which contains high concentrations of the vitamin.

Unpasteurised soft mould-ripened cheese such as Camembert, Brie or chèvre (goats' cheese), blue cheeses and all types of pâté should also be avoided because of the risk of listeria. Tuna, swordfish and marlin contain high levels of mercury, which may damage the unborn baby's nervous system. Make sure you don't eat raw or under-cooked eggs and anything made with them because of the risk of salmonella poisoning.

Is any amount of alcohol safe during pregnancy?

Ideally, it is best to avoid alcohol completely during pregnancy. Studies show that women who drink alcohol while pregnant are more likely to give birth to babies who are smaller, premature or born with abnormalities, including foetal alcohol syndrome. For this reason, the NHS adviser, the National Institute for Health and Clinical Excellence (NICE), advises pregnant women to drink no alcohol, especially in the first three months. It says if they must drink, they should limit their intake to one or two units a week thereafter.

Should I take an omega-3 supplement during pregnancy?

As most of the growth and development of the brain and nervous system takes place before birth (and during the first two years), it is important for pregnant and breast-feeding women to consume plenty of omega-3s. Breast-feeding is important as breast milk supplies omega-3s for babies. Studies show that pregnant women who consume plenty of omega-3 are less likely to give birth to children who suffer from learning and behaviour problems, such as dyslexia, dyspraxia and ADHD (which affects around 1 in 20 children). Research from Purdue University in the US has shown that ADHD children have lower blood concentrations of omega-3 fats.

Do I need extra calcium during pregnancy?

No. The Department of Health does not recommend consuming extra calcium when you are pregnant. Although the baby takes up more calcium during the last trimester as it starts to develop and strengthen its bones, the mother's increased capacity to absorb dietary calcium makes up for this loss without the need for extra intake. The recommended intake for non-pregnant women (700mg) remains unchanged during pregnancy. An extra 500mg a day is recommended during breast-feeding. Dairy products, canned small fish, figs and oranges are good sources of calcium.

- ○ Spinach, broccoli, Brussels sprouts and watercress
- ○ Milk, cheese and yoghurt
- ○ Lean meat, chicken, fish
- ○ Nuts and seeds
- ○ Beans and lentils

Lots of celebrities seem to stay skinny after giving birth – how do they manage it?

Celebrity mums are under pressure to regain their pre-pregnancy skinny figure as fast as possible in order to stay in the limelight. But dieting before, during or immediately after pregnancy isn't healthy for either mother or baby. Getting pregnant while you are dieting can seriously affect your chances of a healthy pregnancy. A 2003 study carried out by Canadian, New Zealand and Australian researchers found that mothers who lose even modest amounts of weight before conceiving risk premature labour, putting their baby's health at risk. Anorexics who do conceive tend to have less healthy babies. And dieting during pregnancy increases the chances of miscarriage, birth complications and having a small-for-date baby, according to studies in New Zealand. It can also result in low intakes of calcium and iron, increasing your chances of brittle bones or iron-deficiency anaemia. Trying to shed your pregnancy weight too quickly after giving birth may result in excessive tiredness, lowered immunity and susceptibility to minor illnesses.

Diet and skin

What should I eat for smoother, younger-looking skin?

Although genetics influences how quickly your skin shows signs of ageing, good nutrition can help minimise the damage and improve the health of your skin. Certain foods play important roles in protecting, regenerating and rehydrating the skin, as well as boosting its smoothness, all of which are vital in slowing down the ageing process. They can't erase wrinkles, but a diet rich in antioxidant nutrients (vitamin C, vitamin E, betacarotene, zinc and selenium) and omega-3 oils will help keep further wrinkles at bay.

A 2001 study by researchers at Monash University, Australia, found that people whose diets are rich in vegetables, fruit, nuts, beans, lentils and wholemeal bread are less likely to wrinkle than those who feast on fatty and sugary foods. More wrinkling was associated with higher intakes of meat (especially processed meats such as sausages and burgers), soft drinks, cakes, pastries, desserts and butter.

Is it true that eating tomatoes stops sunburn?

Eating foods containing high levels of antioxidants will help protect your skin against the damage caused by UV rays, according to researchers. Lycopene, the red pigment found in tomatoes and watermelon, is particularly effective in protecting against sunburn and wrinkles, acting as an internal sunblock. In 2008 researchers at the universities of Manchester and Newcastle found that people who added five tablespoons of tomato paste to their daily diet improved the skin's ability to protect against UV rays by 33 per cent – the equivalent of a low-factor sunscreen. Tomatoes also boosted levels of procollagen in the skin – a molecule that keeps the skin firm. Foods rich in betacarotene, such as mangoes, carrots and apricots, may offer similar protection.

Top ten foods to beat wrinkles

- O Nuts – Most nuts are a good source of selenium, a potent antioxidant that reduces signs of ageing. Brazil nuts contain the most – just two or three a day provide your daily needs.
- O Spinach – Green leafy vegetables such as spinach contain high levels of the antioxidant nutrient lutein, which may help reduce wrinkles as well as prevent age-related eye conditions.
- O Blueberries – Blueberries, as well as raspberries, plums and blackberries, are packed with anthocyanins, which protect against thread veins and help build collagen.
- O Cantaloupe melon – Melons, as well as mangoes, are packed with betacarotene, which promotes healthy new skin cells and boosts the elasticity of the skin.
- O Tomatoes – The lycopene in tomatoes, tomato paste and tomato sauce provide what dermatologists call the 'parasol effect', deflecting some of the UV rays and giving an estimated sun-protection factor of three. However, you should still wear sunscreen at all times in the sun.
- O Peppers – Red, yellow, orange and green peppers have high levels of vitamin C and betacarotene, both of which help keep skin smooth and wrinkle-free.
- O Oats – Oats contain silicic acid, which is needed to make the spongy cells in the skin that lie between collagen and elastin, and help reduce the appearance of lines and wrinkles.
- O Oranges – Oranges and other citrus fruit are full of vitamin C, used in the production of collagen, which keeps the skin looking youthful.

This vitamin also helps strengthen blood capillaries and cell walls.

○ Oily fish – It's a rich source of omega-3 fats, which help keep the walls of the skin cells watertight and ensure the skin stays hydrated.

○ Strawberries – They are packed with ellagic acid, an antioxidant that zaps the free radicals, which when left to rampage around the body break down collagen and elastin in the skin.

Which food should I avoid to prevent wrinkles?

A study at Monash University analysed the diets of 453 elderly people from Australia, Greece and Sweden. The following foods were associated with more wrinkles:

○ Meat, especially processed meats
○ Fast food
○ Butter and hard fats
○ Cakes, biscuits, pastries
○ Desserts
○ Fizzy drinks and cordials

Does chocolate cause breakouts?

Breakouts are usually triggered by stress. But they are also exacerbated by your diet. According to Australian research, eating too many high GI foods – sugary foods and refined starches such as white bread – increases levels of insulin and a hormone called IGF. These cause increased testosterone (yes, even in women) and sebum (oil) production leading to spotty skin. For clearer skin, cut down on processed foods and sugary drinks. Eat instead wholemeal bread and whole-wheat pasta, beans and fresh fruit and vegetables.

Diet and immunity

I often feel run down – what can I eat to boost my immunity?

A poor diet and an unhealthy lifestyle can weaken your immune system, leaving you prone to colds, illnesses and infections. But eating a healthy diet, taking regular moderate exercise and reducing stress levels will help keep your body's immune system healthy and in balance. Most vitamins and minerals are involved in the immune system. The key nutrients include:

Vitamin C – This vitamin is needed by the entire immune system to function normally. For example, interferon, an antiviral chemical secreted by immune cells throughout the body, needs vitamin C for its production. Vitamin C is also used by your body during the healing process, so include plenty of foods rich in this antioxidant. According to a 2007 review of thirty studies by Australian and Finnish researchers involving 11,350 people, taking vitamin C may not protect you from catching a cold but taking extra vitamin C at the beginning of a cold may shorten its duration.

Vitamin A – This vitamin has powerful antioxidant and antiviral properties. It is found in liver, cheese, oily fish, eggs, butter and margarine, and in plant foods in the form of beta-carotene, which the body then converts to vitamin A. Best sources include dark-green vegetables such as spinach and watercress, and yellow, orange and red fruits such as carrots, tomatoes, dried apricots, sweet potatoes and mangoes.

Vitamin E – This vitamin is a powerful antioxidant, which helps keep the immune system healthy. It helps destroy harmful bacteria and fungi. Find it in vegetable oils, margarine, oily fish, nuts, seeds, egg yolk and avocado.

Selenium – This mineral is needed to produce antibodies. Research shows that people with low selenium levels are more likely to succumb to viral infections. Most nuts are good sources of selenium, but Brazil nuts contain especially high levels – just two or three a day will meet your daily requirement.

Zinc – Zinc is involved with the production of certain immune cells – T-cells – whose job it is to seek out, identify and destroy bacteria and viruses. You can find it in eggs, whole-grain cereals, meat, milk and dairy products.

What are the best immunity-boosting foods?

Certain foods can help strengthen your body's defences to prevent illness. Here's how:

Broccoli – Broccoli and other dark-green vegetables such as Brussels sprouts, spinach and curly kale contain high levels of sulforaphane and indoles, strong immune boosters that also help prevent cancer.

Asparagus – This is useful for bolstering your immunity thanks to its content of fructo-oligosaccharides. This type of dietary fibre fuels the healthy types of bacteria in your gut, which keep harmful bugs at bay.

Pomegranates – these contain cancer-fighting polyphenols, immunity-boosting tannins, and anthocyanins, which reduce inflammation and protect blood vessels. They are also rich in vitamins A, C and E, and iron.

Tea – Scientists have shown that protective antioxidant levels rise significantly in the blood within thirty minutes of drinking a cup of tea.

Blackcurrants – All berries contain high levels of anthocyanins, which have antibacterial and antiviral properties. Blueberries and cranberries are particularly good at fighting infection, while blackberries and strawberries are high in vitamin C.

Manuka honey – This honey from New Zealand contains antioxidants, which can help strengthen the immune system and fight infection. All honey is good for soothing sore throats and cold symptoms, and, applied externally, helping cuts and grazes heal faster.

Brazil nuts – Brazils are one of the best sources of the antioxidant mineral selenium which boosts your immune system, as well as helping prevent cancer, heart disease and premature ageing.

Ginger – It contains gingerol oils, which boost the circulation and help fight inflammation, making it useful for fighting colds and flu.

Tomatoes – Tomatoes are full of immunity-boosting vitamin C and lycopene, an antioxidant that helps fight cancer. Cooked tomatoes (e.g. pasta sauce) contain more than raw.

Garlic – Garlic contains allicin, a sulphur-containing compound, which has powerful antibacterial and antiviral properties.

Bio yoghurt – Bio yoghurt, or 'live' yoghurt, contains billions of live or 'friendly' bacteria, which help boost your defence system by triggering the release of immune cells in your body that kill bacteria and viruses.

Oily fish – Oily fish such as salmon, sardines and mackerel are rich in omega-3 fats, which help reduce inflammation and boost overall immunity.

Onions – Onions contain quercetin, a potent flavanoid with antibacterial, anti-inflammatory and antiviral properties, which can help fend off colds and infections.

✳ Immunity boosters

- O All fruit and vegetables – rich in vitamins A, C and E
- O Nuts, whole grains and pulses – rich in zinc, selenium and calcium
- O Oily fish – rich in omega-3 fats
- O Probiotics in live yoghurt and yoghurt drinks
- O Echinacea
- O A good night's sleep
- O Regular moderate exercise
- O A positive mindset; being optimistic
- O Natural daylight
- O Relaxation – try yoga and meditation
- O A good social network

Immunity enemies

- Smoking
- Too much alcohol
- Stress
- Lack of exercise
- Lack of sleep
- Excessive exercise
- Yo-yo dieting

Can echinacea stop me catching a cold?

A 2007 review of studies on echinacea by researchers at the University of Connecticut concluded that this plant extract can help prevent colds, flu and upper respiratory tract infections. Overall, it was shown to decrease the odds of developing a cold by 58 per cent and reduce the duration of colds by a day and a half. It can also reduce the severity of symptoms if you've already caught a cold. Echinacea boosts immunity by stimulating the body's own production of immune cells. Although there are various forms of the supplement available, most of the positive studies have used a tincture.

Are regular exercisers more or less likely to get ill?

More and more research is finding that moderate regular exercise boosts immunity. During exercise immune cells circulate through the body more quickly and are better able to kill bacteria and viruses. This immune boost lasts several hours after exercise. By doing consistent bouts of exercise the immunity benefits become cumulative, resulting in long-term immunity benefits. One study at Appalachian State University found that people who walked briskly for forty minutes daily had half as many sick days due to colds or sore throats as those who didn't exercise. However, too much exercise appears to reduce immunity. It is thought that the increased levels of stress hormones, such as adrenaline and cortisol, associated with intense exercise (more than ninety minutes) inhibit the production of immune cells.

Can dieting weaken my immunity?

It has been shown that yo-yo dieting (repeatedly losing and regaining weight) may weaken the immune system. A 2007 study published in the *Journal of the American Dietetic Association* found that the more times a woman lost weight the greater the decrease in her immune function. Losing weight appears to reduce the activity of 'natural killer cells', which kill viruses and are vital to the immune system.

Diet and tiredness

I sometimes feel tired and lethargic – could this be caused by my diet?

It's not only lack of sleep that can leave you feeling sluggish – bad eating habits also drain your energy levels. If you're generally lacklustre, changing your diet may help boost your vitality. It's worthwhile checking what, how much and when you eat, as they all affect energy levels.

Eating lots of sugar can trigger surges in insulin, which in turn results in blood-sugar dips and low energy levels. Avoid this by cutting down on sugary foods, white bread, white rice and other refined carbs. Choose instead low GI foods such as beans, pasta, fruit and vegetables, which release their energy over a longer period. Combine them with a protein food (chicken, fish, dairy) to reduce the GI further. Divide your daily food intake into three meals and two healthy snacks, which will help maintain blood-sugar levels within a healthy range. Researchers at the Human

Performance Laboratory of Ball State University, US, have shown that eating frequent small meals with a moderate to low GI causes much smaller peaks and troughs in blood sugar and insulin, so creating the ideal environment for glycogen refuelling – and keeping energy levels high. Don't leave long gaps between eating – the resulting hunger may mean you overeat at your next meal, triggering over-production of insulin. Hormone fluctuations during your period can also affect blood-sugar levels, causing tiredness. Include an extra weekly portion of mackerel or salmon in your diet, or take an omega-3 rich supplement. These essential fatty acids help regulate the manufacture and action of hormones and have also been shown to reduce symptoms of PMS.

Does dehydration cause tiredness?

Yes, tiredness can sometimes be caused by dehydration. Losing just 2 per cent of your body weight as fluid – equivalent to 1.2kg in a person weighing 60kg – may result in headache, fatigue, forgetfulness and an elevated heart rate. What's more, dehydration is cumulative and can build over a few days if you don't rehydrate after exercise, for example.

What can I eat to combat a mid-afternoon slump in energy?

If you find yourself nodding off in the afternoons, try adding a little extra protein (chicken, fish or cheese) to your lunch to counteract the sleep-inducing effect of too many carbs. Energy levels naturally dip around 3 p.m. and when this natural dip coincides with a post-lunch blood-sugar dip, you experience an energy slump. Too many carbohydrates trigger a surge of insulin (which causes blood-sugar levels to dip) and serotonin (which make us feel sleepy). So opt for a high-protein, low-carbohydrate lunch, such as a chicken or cheese salad, to increase alertness.

What to eat for boundless energy

- Multigrain, seeded or rye bread – bread with lots of grains or seeds gives a slower energy release than other types. This helps you maintain energy levels throughout the day and avoid energy slumps.
- Bowl of porridge – eating a high-fibre cereal, such as porridge, oat flakes or Shreddies, each day can reduce fatigue by 10 per cent according to a study at a Cardiff University.
- Nuts – these are packed with magnesium, which is vital for energy release in every cell in the body, yet many people's diets are lacking in it. Fatigue is one of the signs of magnesium deficiency. Other sources include whole grains, pumpkin, sunflower and sesame seeds, vegetables and fruit.
- Honey – the main sugar in honey is fructose, which is absorbed more slowly than ordinary sugar, and gives you more sustained energy. Replace sugar in drinks and recipes with honey.
- Sweet potatoes – these are digested more slowly than ordinary potatoes and release their energy more slowly.

Are there any supplements that can give me more energy?

There is little evidence that so-called energy supplements, such as ginseng and coenzyme Q10, boost energy levels. Studies have failed to show that either increases oxygen uptake or endurance. In high doses, ginseng may cause high blood pressure and insomnia. However, coenzyme Q10 is showing promise against Parkinson's disease and also as possible therapy for heart disease patients.

Will energy drinks and energy bars boost my energy?

The term 'energy' in these products refers to the high calorie content of the product. They will not necessarily make you feel more 'energetic'! Energy drinks and bars are intended to be consumed before, during or immediately after vigorous exercise, when they may help boost endurance. They provide a convenient fuel source but offer no significant nutritional advantage over other high-carbohydrate drinks and foods. Some energy drinks claim to increase alertness but this is due to their caffeine content. Check the calorie content on the label – many are high in calories and you may end up consuming more calories than you need.

Diet and PMS

What can I eat to ease the symptoms of PMS?

It is estimated that eight out of ten women experience at least one symptom of Premenstrual Syndrome (PMS). This may include water retention, mood swings, cravings, irritability, acne and stomach cramps. There are several theories about why PMS occurs, but experts believe it is triggered by fluctuations of the sex hormones during the menstrual cycle: a drop in progesterone and an increase in oestrogen in the latter half of the cycle.

There's no proven way to cure it, but making a few changes to your diet can help ease the symptoms:

Eat a healthy diet throughout the month – don't just look at changing your diet in the run-up to your period. Your long-term food intake affects levels of oestrogen, the hormone linked with menstruation. So eating plenty of nutrient-rich foods long-term will help correct any minor nutritional deficiencies, and help reduce hormonal fluctuations responsible for PMS.

Eat little and often – this is beneficial because when blood-sugar levels drop, the body releases adrenaline, which reduces the efficiency of progesterone, the hormone that relieves symptoms of PMS. Avoid skipping meals.

Eat low GI meals – opting for foods that release energy into the blood slowly will help prevent blood-sugar fluctuations. Low blood-sugar levels can make symptoms such as low mood, irritability, cravings and tiredness even worse. Include low GI foods such as whole grains, beans, lentils, fruit, vegetables, yoghurt, milk and nuts.

Eat 'good mood' foods – foods rich in tryptophan will help reduce mood swings and make you feel happier: these include milk, yoghurt, cheese, fish, poultry, meat, lentils, beans, nuts and seeds. The body uses this amino acid to make the feel-good brain chemical, serotonin. For a bigger serotonin boost, eat a tryptophan-rich food along with a carbohydrate-rich food, such as pasta and cheese.

Increase vitamin B6 – this vitamin is involved in making the feel-good hormones serotonin and dopamine, so eating plenty of B6-rich foods will correct any minor deficiency. Good sources include nuts, pulses, eggs, bread, cereals, fish and bananas. There's no proof that B6 supplements cures PMS, but some women find it helps. Avoid doses over 10mg a day, as this may cause numbness and persistent pins and needles in your arms and legs (see page 44 'How much is too much?').

Cut down on salt – too much salt makes the body hold on to extra water, and may aggravate fluid retention. Reduce ready-meals, fast foods, sauces and salty snacks; check labels for their salt content (see page 62 'Salt') and drink more water.

Eat calcium-rich foods – according to a 2006 study at Massachusetts University, women without PMS tend to eat more vitamin D and calcium-rich foods such as milk, cheese, yoghurt and broccoli. Other studies have shown that blood levels of calcium and vitamin D are lower in PMS sufferers. Good sources of vitamin D include sunlight exposure, oily fish and margarine.

Get more magnesium – magnesium is involved in the manufacture of dopamine and serotonin. The American College of Obstetrics and Gynecologists recommends increasing your intake of magnesium to reduce bloating, breast tenderness and mood symptoms. Good sources include whole-grain cereals, fruit, vegetables, nuts and seeds.

Evening primrose oil – this contains the omega-6 essential fatty acid, gamma linoleic acid (GLA), which has anti-inflammatory properties. There is no conclusive proof that it works, but many women find that it reduces breast tenderness and eases menstrual cramps.

Stay active – exercise alleviates painful cramps and boosts your mood.

✳ Foods that help PMS

○ Yoghurt – its high calcium content helps avoid PMS

○ Milk – it's rich in mood-enhancing tryptophan

○ Nuts – contain magnesium to reduce moodiness

○ Beans – low GI foods prevent blood-sugar swings

○ Wholemeal bread – carbohydrates help boost serotonin in the brain

○ Bananas – its vitamin B6 helps PMS

○ Parsley – flavour food with this instead of salt to avoid bloating

○ Herbal tea – helps with fluid retention

○ Evening primrose oil – may reduce breast tenderness

Diet and Food allergy

Are food allergies more common nowadays?

One in three people believes they have an allergy, according to a 2002 Datamonitor survey – but less than 2 per cent actually do. Studies have shown that many people self-diagnose food allergies.

What causes a food allergy?

A food allergy is caused when the body mistakenly makes an antibody (IgE) to 'fight off' a specific food. The body sees the food as a foreign substance and mounts an attack against it by producing IgE antibodies. When the food is next eaten (or comes into contact with the skin) it triggers an immune system response, which results in the release of histamine and other chemicals in the body. Reactions include swelling lips, vomiting and diarrhoea, itching and swelling, or a runny nose or sneezing. The foods that most commonly cause food allergy are milk, eggs, nuts, seeds, shellfish, fish, wheat, soya, strawberries and citrus fruit.

What is the difference between a food allergy and food intolerance?

A true food allergy involves the immune system and produces symptoms instantly after the food is eaten or touched. On the other hand, a food intolerance – which is much more common – does not involve the immune system. Symptoms are usually slower to develop and may last several hours. It is a reaction to a food caused by the body's inability to break down or digest that food. This can lead to symptoms such as migraine, bloating and aches and pains. It is not as serious or life-threatening as an allergy.

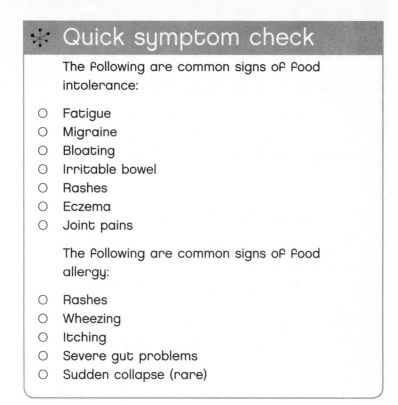

I think I may have an allergy – what should I do?

If you think that you have an allergy or an intolerance you should contact your GP and ask for a referral to your nearest allergy specialist. They may carry out one of the following tests:

Blood Test: This test measures the amount of specific IgE circulating in the blood that the immune system has produced against a suspected allergen.

Skin Prick Testing: This test involves pricking the skin and adding a suspected allergen. If a small red weal appears, you know it's a problem allergen. It measures specific IgE attached to cells in the skin important in allergies called 'mast' cells. The test is conducted within a hospital or GP surgery by specially trained nurses or doctors.

Elimination and Challenge Test: This is usually used for diagnosing food intolerances. It involves eliminating the suspected food(s) and then reintroducing them to see whether symptoms reappear. Ideally, you should see a dietitian who will provide an elimination diet tailored to your specific needs.

Other tests: Other tests include food challenge tests where you are given the suspected substance. It could, of course, trigger an allergic reaction, so should only be done at a specialist hospital clinic.

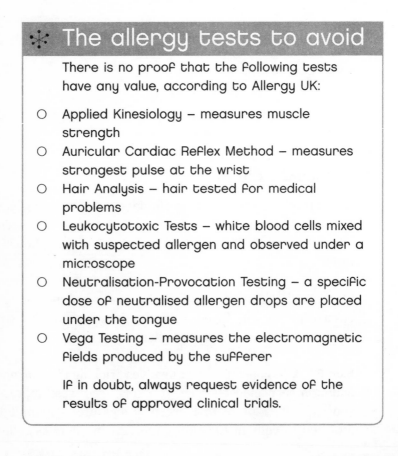

✳ The allergy tests to avoid

There is no proof that the following tests have any value, according to Allergy UK:

○ Applied Kinesiology – measures muscle strength
○ Auricular Cardiac Reflex Method – measures strongest pulse at the wrist
○ Hair Analysis – hair tested for medical problems
○ Leukocytotoxic Tests – white blood cells mixed with suspected allergen and observed under a microscope
○ Neutralisation-Provocation Testing – a specific dose of neutralised allergen drops are placed under the tongue
○ Vega Testing – measures the electromagnetic fields produced by the sufferer

If in doubt, always request evidence of the results of approved clinical trials.

Can my food allergies be cured?

Once you have found the cause of your symptoms, the only treatment is to avoid the offending food(s). There are no cures for allergy or intolerance. You have to avoid the foods that cause your allergy totally. If you have a severe allergy it is crucial that you don't eat (or touch in some cases) even minute amounts of that food.

Chapter 5

Diet and Health

W e've seen the effects that our diet can have on the way we feel, from combating stress and tiredness to boosting brain power and immunity.

But when it comes to dodging major diseases, the evidence is stronger than ever that our food can play a major role. Whether it's heart disease, diabetes or cancer, there's mounting evidence that we can significantly reduce our risk of contracting certain illnesses by switching to a healthier diet and by doing more exercise.

In other words, changing the way we lead our life can have a massive impact on our health. This chapter gives you the low-down on four preventable diseases and what you can do to avoid getting them.

Diet and heart disease

Heart disease is the main cause of death in the UK – 2.6 million people are affected by it and, in 2004, 216,000 people died from it, accounting for about 37 per cent of all deaths. Smoking, being overweight, having a high level of cholesterol in your blood, high blood pressure, diabetes, stress and being physically inactive all increase your chances of developing heart disease or stroke. But . . .

How does diet help prevent heart disease?

What you eat may reduce your chances of developing heart disease by:

○ Keeping your weight in the healthy range
○ Lowering your blood pressure
○ Lowering levels of 'bad' LDL cholesterol
○ Increasing levels of 'good' cholesterol
○ Preventing blood clots that can lead to heart attack and stroke

A healthy diet can also increase your chances of survival after suffering a heart attack.

What's the biggest thing I can do to cut my heart disease risk?

Maintaining a healthy stable weight is one of the most important ways of reducing your heart disease risk. Being overweight puts strain on your organs, including your heart. It is estimated that overweight and physical inactivity together account for two thirds of deaths from cardiovascular disease. Having a body mass index (BMI) greater than 25 (see page 86, 'What is my BMI?') greatly increases your chance of developing diabetes, high blood cholesterol and high blood pressure – all of which make it more likely that you will develop heart disease (see page 89 'I'm not ill now so is it really unhealthy to be overweight?').

If you are already at a healthy weight, aim to keep your BMI within a healthy range of 18.5 to 24.9. Gaining as little as 5kg during adulthood can significantly increase your risk of heart disease, diabetes and high blood pressure – no matter how slim you were earlier in your life.

I have a bit of a paunch but have slim legs and arms. My doctor tells me I'm risking my health – why?

Having excess fat around your waist ('apple-shaped' obesity) is considered a big risk factor for heart disease. The problem with this type of fat is that it has easier access to the blood supply of the liver. It increases the liver's production of very low-density lipoproteins and reduces its sensitivity to insulin (which increases the risk of type 2 diabetes). These changes increase the risk of heart disease, and also other metabolic complications. A simple way to measure whether you are 'apple-shaped' is to measure your waist circumference. It should be less than 80cm (32 inches) in women, and less than 94cm (37 inches) in men.

What is a high blood cholesterol level?

A high blood cholesterol level is judged to be above 5.0 mmol/l, according to the National Institute for Health and Clinical Excellence (NICE). Usually, when you have your blood cholesterol measured, your GP will look at your total cholesterol level, plus your LDL and HDL cholesterol (see page 42, 'What does LDL and HDL cholesterol mean?') Healthy levels of cholesterol are:

O   Total cholesterol – below 5 mmol/l
O   LDL cholesterol – below 3 mmol/l
O   HDL cholesterol – above 1 mmol/l

Are there any specific foods that will lower my cholesterol levels?

Canadian researchers found that when people with high cholesterol levels consumed at least four daily portions of foods containing soluble fibre, soy, almonds and plant sterols, their cholesterol levels dropped by an average 14 per cent after 12 weeks. And, according the 2006 study, eating cholesterol-lowering foods can cut cholesterol levels as effectively as taking statins (cholesterol-lowering drugs). Those who stuck to the diet most closely cut their cholesterol by more than 20 per cent, similar to that seen with drugs.

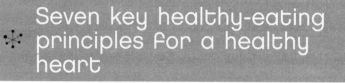

Seven key healthy-eating principles for a healthy heart

1. Eat 'good' fats instead of 'bad' fats
2. Get plenty of fruit and vegetables
3. Eat a Mediterranean-style diet
4. Eat more fibre
5. Control your weight
6. Cut down on salt
7. Stick to healthy alcohol limits

Is a low-fat diet healthier for my heart?

Despite popular belief, a low-fat diet is not necessarily the healthiest one for your heart. Much evidence now points to the benefits of eating a diet containing moderate – around 35 per cent of calories from fat – rather than low levels of fat. A 2004 study at New York State University found that people on a moderate-fat diet had healthier blood-cholesterol levels than those following a low-fat regime. The reason, suggest the researchers, is because most of the fats on the moderate-fat diet were the monounsaturated kind, including nuts and olive oil. Another study in 2008 also found that people who ate a moderately high-fat diet containing plenty of monounsaturated fat for six months lowered their risk of diabetes and blood-insulin levels, both major risk factors for heart disease. Experts now believe that the total amount of fat in your diet may not matter at all – it's the kind of fats you eat that matters most for your heart health.

So which fats should I be eating?

Focus on replacing 'bad' fats with 'good' ones. The bad fats are saturated and trans fat, which increase 'bad' LDL cholesterol (see page 33), the kind that builds up on artery walls. Trans fats also reduce 'good' HDL cholesterol (see page 42) and increase levels of blood fats (triglycerides), both important risk factors for heart disease.

The 'good' fats are unsaturated fats, including the monounsaturates and polyunsaturates (see page 36). They're found in nuts, seeds, olives (and their oils) and fish. Eating 'good' fats instead of saturated and trans fats can protect your heart because it raises HDL cholesterol and lowers LDL cholesterol levels. The Department of Health recommends that, while you should get a maximum of 33 per cent of your calories from fat, only one third of those should come from saturated fat. The majority should come from unsaturated fat, including at least 0.9g of omega-3s per day.

The Guideline Daily Amount (GDA) for total fat and saturated fat

	Men	Women
Fat	95g	70g
Saturated fat	30g	20g

How do omega-3s cut my heart attack risk?

There is plenty of evidence to suggest that people with the highest intakes of omega-3s have the lowest risk of heart disease and stroke. Omega-3s can help reduce the stickiness of the blood, making it less likely to clot. They also help the blood flow more easily through the smallest blood vessels, reduce blood-fat (triglycerides) levels and help raise HDL cholesterol levels, which protect against heart attacks. You should aim to consume 0.9g of omega-3 daily, an amount that can be obtained from one portion (140g) of oily fish eaten once a week (sardines, mackerel, salmon, fresh (not tinned) tuna, trout and herring), 15g of walnuts or pumpkin seeds, one teaspoon of flaxseed oil, one tablespoon of rapeseed oil or soya oil, or two omega-3 eggs.

I know that fruit and vegetables are good for me but will they reduce my chances of heart disease?

Fruit and vegetables are packed with antioxidants, which help protect against heart disease. These include betacarotene, vitamin C and flavanoids, as well as hundreds of other phytonutrients. Antioxidants mop up free radicals (see page 53), which can cause oxidation of LDL cholesterol and 'furring' of the arteries. In their 2003 report, *Diet, Nutrition and the Prevention of Chronic Disease*, the World Health Organisation stated that there was convincing evidence that eating 400g (five portions) of fruit and vegetables a day decreases the risk of heart disease. Several studies have linked a high intake of flavanoids – found mainly in fruit, vegetables and nuts – with a low rate of heart disease. Flavanoids are powerful antioxidants and have also been shown to reduce the likelihood of clots forming.

A 2008 study by the Finnish National Public Health Institute showed that eating berries, rich in flavanoids, reduced platelet stickiness, increased HDL cholesterol and lowered blood pressure. Vitamin C-rich fruit also helps reduce furring of the arteries, according to a 2008 study by Norwegian researchers.

What's all the fuss about folic acid?

Much recent research on heart disease has focused on folic acid. That's because it has been shown to reduce blood levels of homocysteine, an amino acid that is a natural by-product of the breakdown of protein. Raised homocysteine levels in the blood damage the cells that line the arteries, increasing heart disease risk. The good news is that upping your intake of folate – a B-vitamin found in green leafy vegetables, whole grains, beans, lentils and liver – reduces your heart disease risk.

Will switching to a Mediterranean diet stop me getting a heart attack?

A traditional Mediterranean-style diet emphasises fruit and vegetables, oily fish, low amounts of red meat and dairy foods, plenty of whole grains, beans, nuts and seeds, olive oil as a source of fat, and small amounts of wine. Studies across a number of countries have shown that people who follow this type of diet have a lower rate of heart disease and strokes and live longer. In general, they consume less saturated fat and more monounsaturated fats.

A 2003 study of 2,200 people by researchers at the University of Athens showed that the closer their eating habits matched the Mediterranean diet, the lower their heart disease risk. Researchers measured lower levels of a substance called C-reactive protein in their blood, a marker of inflammation related to heart disease. Another study, the Lyon Diet Heart Study, published in 2001, looked at the diets of 600 heart attack survivors. After four years, those following a Mediterranean-style diet had a 50 to 70 per cent lower risk of recurrent heart disease.

Is too much meat bad for my heart?

Quite possibly. Red meat is a major source of saturated fat in the average person's diet, and has been linked to an increased heart disease risk. For example, US researchers found that people who eat two or more servings of red meat a day are more likely to develop conditions leading to heart disease. The 2008 study carried out at the University of Minnesota found people who ate more than two portions of red meat per week were 25 per cent more likely to have excessive fat around the waist, high cholesterol, high blood sugar and high blood pressure – a cluster of risk factors known as metabolic syndrome – than those who ate fewer than two weekly portions.

I know that a high-fibre diet is often promoted for weight loss – can it also benefit my heart?

Eating more fibre has numerous health benefits. But it's the soluble type of fibre, found in oats, beans, lentils, fruit and vegetables (see page 23: 'What is fibre?') that is a great ally in keeping your heart healthy. It helps by reducing the amount of cholesterol absorbed from the intestines, thus helping lower levels of cholesterol in the blood and reducing the risk of heart disease.

Soluble fibre also helps slow the digestion and absorption of carbohydrates, reducing blood sugar and insulin levels. High levels of blood insulin are associated with a higher heart disease risk.

✳ Bananas and blood cholesterol

Bananas may help keep your cholesterol levels in check. That's because under-ripe bananas contain a type of fibre, called resistant starch, which may reduce the risk of heart disease (see page 26 'I've heard of "resistant starch" – is it the same as fibre?'). It's also found in beans and lentils and it's useful in your battle against heart disease because it passes unchanged into the large intestine. Here, it is fermented by your 'friendly' gut bacteria, which produce short-chain fatty acids. These fatty acids are absorbed into the bloodstream and help lower blood-cholesterol levels.

There are lots of soya products that claim to help reduce cholesterol levels – do they work?

Soya contains soluble fibre as well as chemical compounds called isoflavones, which have a positive impact on cholesterol levels. They are natural compounds that mimic the effects of oestrogen in the body and as a result will raise HDL levels. Studies have shown that including at least 25g of soya in your daily diet, provided it is low in saturated fat, reduces blood cholesterol. You can get this amount of soya by drinking three glasses of soya milk.

Do products containing plant sterols work?

Yes, but only if you have high blood-cholesterol levels to start with and you eat enough of them! Plant sterols or phytosterols have a similar structure to human cholesterol. They occur naturally in many vegetable oils, including soya, rapeseed, corn and sunflower oil as well as nuts and seeds. They are also added to spreads, yoghurt drinks, milks and yoghurts. Popular brand names include Flora Pro-active, Benecol and Danone Danacol. Plant sterols work by blocking the absorption of cholesterol from the intestines, thus reducing LDL cholesterol levels in the bloodstream. You can expect a cholesterol reduction of around 10 to 14 per cent if you consume around 2g per day, according to a 2005 study at the Maastricht University in the Netherlands. Less than this amount probably won't provide much benefit, according to a 2004 study at Washington University. You can get 2g from a 100ml one-shot yoghurt drink, or a 125ml pot of (sterol) yoghurt, or two glasses of (sterol) milk or two servings of sterol spread. The FSA cautions against more than 3g daily.

How can cutting salt stop me getting heart disease?

Eating too much salt can cause raised blood pressure, which triples the risk of heart disease and stroke (see page 62 'We're told to cut down on salt – why?'). Having high blood pressure means your heart has to work harder to push the blood around your body. And this extra pressure puts extra strain on your arteries that carry the blood, which can weaken. The Food Standards Agency estimates that the resulting falls in blood pressure between 2001 and 2008 when the average salt intake fell from 9.5g to 8.6g prevented 7,000 heart attack and stroke deaths in the UK. Cutting salt to 6g would lead to a further 10 per cent drop in heart disease cases.

Three quarters of the salt in the average diet comes from processed foods. Check the labels of food for salt and aim to consume no more than 6g daily.

✴ How to cut salt

○ Avoid foods containing more than 1.25g salt per 100g

○ Don't add salt to cooking or at the table

○ Buy 'low salt' versions of everyday foods, such as bread, cereal and tinned foods

○ Use herbs and spices such as garlic, oregano and lemon juice to add flavour to meals

○ Limit salty foods such as ready-meals, burgers, sausages, pizza, takeaways, sauces and savoury packet snacks

Is a daily tipple good for my heart?

According to the British Heart Foundation, drinking one or two units of alcohol daily may protect against heart disease. In moderation, alcohol helps raise HDL levels and reduces the tendency for platelets to clump together and form clots (see page 69 'I'm confused about alcohol – is it beneficial or harmful?'). However, the studies to support this recommendation involved men over the age of forty and post-menopausal women – the benefits for other people are not proven. Red wine in particular appears the most cardio-protective due to its high content of polyphenols, saponins and a compound called resveratrol.

The UK Department of Health advises a maximum of three units a day and fourteen units a week for women, and a maximum of four units daily and twenty-one units weekly for men. One unit is half a pint of beer or a 125ml glass of 8 per cent ABV wine (see page 70 'What's a unit?'). Drinking more than these levels increases your health risk.

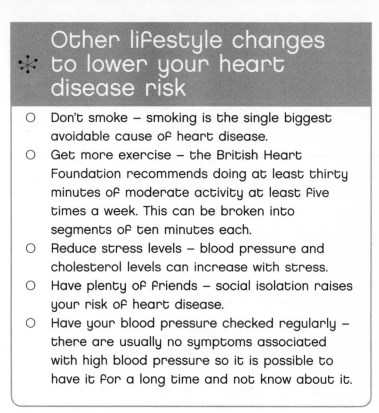

Diet and cancer

Around one in three people in the UK develops cancer at some point during their lifetime. But there is a huge amount of research that shows you can reduce your cancer risk by changing what you eat, being more active and maintaining a healthy weight. The largest review of links between diet and cancer, incorporating the findings of 7,000 research studies from all over the world, was published by the World Cancer Research Fund (WCRF) in 2007. It concluded that there is convincing evidence that diet plays a role in many cancers.

Seven key healthy-eating principles to cut your cancer risk

Experts say that by following these recommendations of the WCRF report you could reduce your risk of cancer by about a third:

1. Stay lean
2. Avoid calorie-dense foods
3. Eat more fruit, vegetables, whole grains and pulses
4. Don't eat much meat
5. Don't drink much alcohol
6. Cut salt
7. Make time for daily exercise

What is the single biggest thing I can do that will cut my cancer risk?

Maintaining a healthy weight – ideally at the lower end of the recommended range for your height – is the most important step you can take to reduce your cancer risk. Being even slightly overweight increases your risk of a range of common cancers, including bowel, breast, pancreatic and kidney cancer. Cancer Research UK found that breast cancer risk can be as much as double in post-menopausal women who are overweight. It's likely to be because fat cells release hormones such as oestrogen, which increase the risk of breast cancer. But fat stored around the waist is the most risky because it encourages the body to produce 'growth hormones' that make cancer cells grow.

The WCRF advises being at the lower end of the healthy weight range, or 'as lean as possible without becoming underweight'. This might sound difficult, but this is what the science is saying more clearly than ever. Putting on weight can increase your cancer risk, even if you are within the healthy range. A healthy weight is defined as having a BMI below 25 (see page 86, 'What is my BMI?').

A healthy waist measurement is less than 80cm (32 inches) for women and less than 94cm (37 inches) for men.

So many foods have been linked with cancer – which ones are the worst culprits?

The WCRF considers processed meat, red meat, sugary foods, sugary drinks and foods high in saturated fat the biggest culprits when it comes to cancer risk.

The 2005 European Prospective Investigation into Cancer and Nutrition (EPIC) study, which looked at the eating habits of over 500,000 people across Europe over 10 years, found that the more meat you eat, the greater the risk of bowel cancer. A 2001 study by the Human Nutrition Unit at Cambridge University showed that eating lots of red meat creates as many carcinogens in the colon as smoking does in the lungs. Haem compounds found in red meat trigger the formation of carcinogenic (cancer-causing) N-nitroso compounds in the gut. About 500g (five palm-sized portions) of red meat (beef, lamb and pork) a week is fine, but more than that might increase your risk of bowel cancer, according to the WRCF.

Processed meat always gets a bad press, but can sausages really cause cancer?

The WCRF report states that eating just 50g a day of processed meat, such as sausages, bacon and ham, increases your cancer risk by 21 per cent. They recommend cutting out all processed meats. The problem is the nitrates in the meats, which lead to the formation of carcinogens in your bowel. But salt, which is often added to processed meats, may also play a role. It may promote inflammation in the stomach, which can lead to cancer. Stick to less than 6g of salt a day (see page 63 'How much salt should I have, then?'). Cured and smoked meats also contain carcinogens, substances that can damage body cells and lead to cancer.

Do sugar and fat also increase my chances of cancer?

Foods that are high in saturated fat, sugar and calories increase the risk of weight gain and obesity, which in turn increases the chances of developing a range of cancers including bowel and breast cancer. A 2003 Canadian study involving 580,000 women found that eating lots of fatty foods, particularly those high in saturated fat, increases the risk of breast cancer by 20 per cent.

But the WCRF report warns against sugary drinks in particular. The problem is they don't promote satiety (see page 104) or subsequent compensation in calorie intake, and so encourage overconsumption of calories and weight gain.

The WCRF recommends cutting down on foods with a calorie density greater than 225 to 275kcal per 100g (see box 'Cancer and diet' page 185). The exceptions include foods such as nuts, avocados, olive oil and seeds, which are packed with nutrients, so should be eaten in smaller portions rather than eliminated.

Focus on foods with a low calorie density, in other words, foods that contain relatively few calories per gram. These foods contain plenty of fibre and water, less fat and/ or sugar, and provide maximum filling power for fewest calories. They help control your appetite and stave off hunger pangs.

Cancer and diet

Avoid calorie-dense foods	Eat more low calorie-dense foods
Cakes, biscuits, puddings	Fruit
Fast foods – burgers, sausages, chips, pizzas, nuggets	Vegetables
	Salad
Takeaways and ready-meals	Beans and lentils
Crisps and packet snacks	Whole grains e.g. wholemeal bread, whole-wheat pasta, oats, whole-grain breakfast cereals and brown rice
Chocolate	
Sweets	
Butter	
Bacon	Low-fat milk and yoghurt
Roast or fried meat	

Are there any foods that could protect me from cancer?

Eating at least five portions of fruit and vegetables a day is a major protection factor. These foods protect against a wide range of cancers including mouth, stomach, lung, prostate and pancreatic cancer. As well as containing vitamins and minerals, which strengthen the immune system, fruit and vegetables are also good sources of phytonutrients. These are plant compounds that help to protect body cells from damage that can lead to cancer.

According to the WCRF report, foods rich in fibre decrease the risk of bowel cancer. It recommends eating whole grains or pulses (beans and lentils) with every meal. The US dietary guidelines recommend a minimum of three servings of whole-grain foods a day. One serving is one slice of wholemeal bread or a third of a cup of whole-wheat pasta.

The 2003 'EPIC' study by Cancer Research UK and the Medical Research Council involving more than half a million people in ten European countries found a clear link between the amount of fibre eaten and the incidence of bowel cancer – those with least fibre in their diets had the biggest risk of bowel cancer. A 2007 study at the University of Leeds found that women eating 30g of fibre a day halved their risk of breast cancer compared with low fibre eaters (less than 20g).

But certain vegetables are particularly protective against cancer. These include broccoli, cabbage and cauliflower, which contain indole-3-carbinol and genistein. These compounds boost the body's ability to repair damaged DNA and may prevent cells turning cancerous, according to a 2006 study from Georgetown University in Washington DC.

✳ Mediterranean diet cuts cancer

Adopting a Mediterranean diet may cut your cancer risk. Researchers have found that people living in countries such as Spain and Greece where they generally eat more vegetables and fish, less red meat, cook in olive oil and drink moderate amounts of alcohol, have lower rates of cancer. A 2008 study of 26,000 Greek people found that eating less meat and more pulses cut the risk of cancer by 12 per cent. Using more olive oil alone cut the risk by 9 per cent.

Any other cancer-fighting foods I should eat?

Including nuts and pulses in your diet will help cut your cancer risk, too. According to a 2005 study by the University of London, these foods are rich in a compound, inositol pentakisphosphate, which has been shown to inhibit the growth of tumours. In its dietary guidelines for 2005, the US Department of Agriculture recommends people eat the equivalent of three cups of beans a week.

Selenium, which can be found in Brazil nuts, may help the body defend itself against breast cancer and other types of cancer. Scientists from the University of Illinois found that this mineral helps the body's 'cancer-fighting' enzymes work properly and recommended that women may benefit from extra selenium in their diet.

✳ The anti-cancer diet

What to avoid	What to eat
Ham, bacon, pastrami, salami, hot dogs, sausages – strongly linked to bowel cancer.	Broccoli and Brussels sprouts – contain sulphoraphane, which protects against cancer.
Fast foods, biscuits, cakes – high-fat and sugar foods are linked with obesity and several cancers.	Carrots, tomatoes, mangoes – contain betacarotene, which helps the immune system combat cancer.
Smoked, cured and barbecued food – linked to stomach and oesophagus cancer.	Beans, lentils, wholemeal bread, brown rice and whole-wheat pasta – for fibre, aim to get three portions a day.
Fizzy drinks, squash, cordial – the WCRF warns against sugary drinks.	Sardines, mackerel, herring, salmon – good substitutes for meat; contain omega-3 fats which fight cancer.
	Brazil nuts – contain cancer-fighting selenium.
	Soya milk/ yoghurt – a rich source of phyto-oestrogens, which may block the cancer-causing effect of your own oestrogen.

Will alcohol increase or decrease my cancer risk?

Alcohol has been linked to increased risk of breast, liver, mouth, oesophagus and bowel cancers because it can damage DNA, increasing the risk of cancer. Carcinogens are formed when the body breaks down alcohol. It is estimated that each drink you have daily increases your risk of breast cancer by 7 per cent. The WCRF recommends, ideally, not drinking alcohol at all, but if you must drink then limiting your consumption to no more than two units a day for men and one unit for women. One unit is half a pint of beer or a 125ml glass of 8 per cent ABV wine (see page 70 'What's a unit?').

A 2008 study from the Breast Institute and St George's Hospital, London, suggests that the 5 per cent increase in breast cancer observed over the last ten years is due to the 40 per cent rise in women's drinking. But binge drinking is twice as dangerous for your health as the same amount drunk over a week, according to Danish research. This 2007 study found that women who drank more than four units in one day or ten units over a weekend had more than double the risk of breast cancer, because high alcohol intake increases levels of oestrogen.

To reduce your risk of cancer, you should limit the amount of alcohol you drink and avoid consuming more than four units in one day.

✳ Salt and stomach cancer

Consuming too much salt is believed to cause stomach cancer. Studies have shown that high salt intakes can damage the lining of the stomach, which increases the chances of cancer. Limit your salt intake to 6g daily by cutting down on processed foods, especially bacon, ham, sausages, sauces, ready-meals and crisps (see page 63 'What's the easiest way to cut down on salt?').

What else can I do to reduce my chances of cancer?

Regular exercise protects against bowel and breast cancers because it reduces levels of hormones that cancers need to grow, such as oestrogen and insulin growth factor. The WCRF report recommends exercising for at least thirty minutes a day, but the more you do and the harder you work, the greater the protection.

Getting a daily fifteen-minute dose of sunshine (even in the winter months) will ensure you get enough vitamin D, which may help protect you from cancer. Most of the vitamin D in the body is created during skin exposure to UV light, but can also be obtained from oily fish, margarine and egg yolk. Several studies have linked low blood levels of vitamin D with an increased risk of developing breast, ovarian and colon cancer. A 2005 review of 63 studies by researchers at the University of California concluded that vitamin D could reduce the risk by as much as 50 per cent. Some experts believe that the RDA for vitamin D should be increased from 200IU to 800–1,000IU.

Protecting your skin from UV rays – even on cloudy days – is essential, not only to avoid painful sunburn but also to cut your risk of skin cancer. Sunburn can double your risk of skin cancer, the most common cancer in the UK with around 60,000 new cases each year. Melanoma is the deadliest form and is triggered by sunlight.

If you have fair skin that burns or freckles easily, or you have red or fair hair and blue or green eyes, or you have lots of moles, you need to be extra careful. Wear sunscreen – at least factor 15 and one that offers 4-star protection from UVA.

Diet and diabetes

Over 2 million people, nearly 1 in 20, in the UK have diabetes and a further half a million have it but don't know it. It is a condition where the body cannot convert glucose in the blood into energy because the hormone insulin is not produced. Diabetes is a serious condition, which, if left untreated, can lead to heart disease, blindness, kidney failure and other life-threatening complications. Not many people realise that having type 2 diabetes can reduce your life expectancy by up to ten years. Fortunately, if you spot the symptoms early you can reduce your chances of serious problems.

What is the difference between type 1 and type 2 diabetes?

Type 1 diabetes develops if the body is unable to produce any insulin and is treated with regular insulin injections, diet and physical activity. It usually affects people under forty. Type 2 diabetes develops when the body can still make some insulin, but not enough, or when the insulin that is produced does not work properly (insulin resistance). It is usually associated with being overweight and is found mostly in adults – although an increasing number of children are being diagnosed with the condition. It can be treated with diet and physical activity, although you may also need tablets or injections.

✳ Diabetes symptoms

- Increased thirst
- Going to the toilet all the time – especially at night
- Extreme tiredness
- Weight loss
- Blurred vision
- Genital itching or regular episodes of thrush
- Slow healing of wounds

How do I know whether I am at risk of diabetes?

More than 80 per cent of people with type 2 diabetes are overweight. The more overweight and the more inactive you are, the greater your risk. Excess fat around the waist also puts you at high risk. A waist measurement more than 80cm (32 inches) in women or more than 94cm (37 inches) in men puts you at increased risk of diabetes. Other risk factors include:

○ Having type 2 diabetes in your family
○ High blood pressure, or heart attack or stroke
○ Polycystic ovary syndrome and overweight
○ Impaired glucose tolerance or impaired fasting glycaemia (high level of blood sugar)
○ A history of gestational (pregnancy) diabetes

What is the single biggest step I can take to avoid diabetes?

The single most important step you can take is not being overweight, or to lose weight if you are overweight. Switching to a diet low in saturated fat and sugar, eating plenty of fruit and vegetables, and taking regular exercise will help reduce your risk. In 2005 researchers at the University of California demonstrated a link between a high-fat diet and type 2 diabetes. Another US study in 2004 found that eating lots of refined carbohydrates and too little fibre can cause diabetes.

Can diabetes be treated?

Type 1 diabetes is treated by insulin injections as well as a healthy diet and regular exercise. People with this type of diabetes usually take two or four injections of insulin each day.

Type 2 diabetes is treated with lifestyle changes such

as a healthier diet, weight loss and increased physical activity. Tablets and/or insulin may also be required to achieve normal blood-glucose levels in some people. The main aim of treatment of both types of diabetes is to achieve blood glucose, blood pressure and cholesterol levels as near to normal as possible. This, together with a healthy lifestyle, will help to improve your health and protect against long-term damage to the eyes, kidneys, nerves, heart and major arteries.

Do diabetics need to follow a special diet?

Healthy eating advice for people with diabetes is no different than the advice for everyone else. You do not need to eat special foods or meals. Essentially, you should eat plenty of high-fibre carbohydrate foods such as whole-grain breads and cereals, and vegetables and fruit; and limit your fat intake, especially saturated fat. In fact, eating a Mediterranean-style diet (see page 176) can lower your risk of developing diabetes in the first place by 83 per cent, according to a 2008 Spanish study. The aim of your diet is to control blood-glucose levels, achieve normal blood-lipid (fat) levels, maintain a healthy blood pressure, maintain a healthy weight and prevent or slow the development of diabetes complications.

Basic eating guidelines:

○ Eat regular meals throughout the day.
○ You may need to limit the serving size of your meals and snacks, as too much food will lead to an increase in body weight.
○ Include a high-carbohydrate food at each meal, opting for low GI carbohydrates wherever possible – grainy bread, pasta, Basmati rice, sweet potatoes.
○ Include beans, lentils and oats – these low GI foods help maintain blood-sugar levels.
○ Select a variety of healthy foods from the different food groups.

- Reduce saturated fats e.g. full-fat dairy products, meat fats (trim the fat from meat and limit your intake of processed meats), fried foods, cakes, pastries and foods containing palm oil and coconut oil.
- Include unsaturated fats such as olive or sunflower oil, mono- or polyunsaturated margarines, oily fish, avocado, seeds and nuts.
- Reduce the amount of sugar in your diet – but you don't have to cut out sugar completely; the sugar you do eat should be eaten in nutritious foods such as breakfast cereals or yoghurt rather than sweets or cakes.
- Avoid sugary drinks – sugar in drinks is more rapidly absorbed than sugar in food.
- Don't add salt to your food, and cut down on salty foods.
- Limit alcohol to 21 units weekly for men and 14 units weekly for women. Have at least two alcohol-free days per week.

As a diabetic, should I carry dextrose tablets around?

Only people on insulin need to carry and use sugary snacks when they are going hypo. Generally people with type 2 diabetes will not go hypo and do not need such precautions.

Does eating too much sugar cause diabetes?

No, eating sugar does not cause diabetes. Diabetes is caused by a combination of genetic and environmental factors. However, eating a diet high in fat and sugar can cause you to become overweight, which increases your risk of developing type 2 diabetes, so if you have a history of diabetes in your family, a healthy diet and regular exercise are recommended to control your weight.

Can people with diabetes play sport?

Definitely! There are many successful sportspeople who are diabetic – including Steve Redgrave, Olympic gold medal-winning rower. You should aim to be as active as possible. Try to do at least thirty minutes of moderate-intensity physical activity most days and make the most of other opportunities to be active. Keeping active can help avoid complications associated with diabetes, such as heart disease. There may be some considerations to take into account with your diabetes before taking up a new exercise regime – talk to your healthcare team for more information.

Diet and osteoporosis

One in two women and one in five men aged over fifty in the UK develop osteoporosis, but the good news is the right diet and exercise programme can help reduce the likelihood of you getting the condition. Osteoporosis means just what its name suggests – porous bones (or thinning of the bones). The condition occurs because from around the age of thirty-five more bone cells are lost than replaced, so bone density decreases. The most important thing is to make your bones as strong as possible while you're young. If this is high, you'll have greater bone reserves to help you face the natural loss of ageing. This can be achieved through a calcium-rich diet and regular weight-bearing exercise.

Why are women more likely than men to develop osteoporosis?

Women are especially prone to the disease due to loss of oestrogen after the menopause. During this time, bone loss speeds up, making osteoporosis more likely. In women the risk is increased if they have an early menopause, have their ovaries removed before the menopause, or miss periods for six months or more as a result of excessive exercising or dieting. For men, low levels of testosterone increase the risk. Osteoporosis may cause people to 'shrink' as they get older. It causes the characteristic 'dowager's hump'.

How do I know if I have osteoporosis?

There may be no warning before a minor bump or fall causes a bone fracture, which may result in pain, disability and loss of independence, or even prove fatal. Screening tests – usually involving a bone density scan – exist, although you may have to pay for them privately. This painless test involves a low dose of x-rays (less than a normal x-ray), usually across your spine, wrist or hip. The specialist will then tell you whether you have osteoporosis, or are at risk, and will suggest treatments.

✳ Am I at risk?

- ○ Absence of periods, early menopause or hysterectomy
- ○ Infrequent periods (especially linked to anorexia or excessive exercise)
- ○ Family history of osteoporosis, easy fractures or dowager's hump
- ○ Use of corticosteroids
- ○ Being underweight
- ○ Little regular physical activity
- ○ High intake of alcohol
- ○ Smoking
- ○ Low testosterone levels in men

How can diet prevent osteoporosis?

Research suggests that getting enough calcium and vitamin D will help maximise your potential bone density, but taking extra (more than the RDA) won't necessarily prevent osteoporosis in adults. However, studies have shown that when children and teenagers consume extra calcium, such as extra dairy products or calcium supplements, their bone density increases in the short term. But not many studies have measured bone density for longer periods. Whether this extra bone mass continues into adulthood is not known.

Despite popular belief, high intakes of calcium seem to have no effect in preventing bone loss during and immediately after the menopause. Experts recommend hormone replacement therapy (HRT) to prevent bone loss around the menopause. Calcium and Vitamin D supplements may help reduce bone loss (particularly in the hip) and fracture risk in older people.

✳ Kick the cola habit for stronger bones

Drinking cola and other fizzy drinks can lower your bone density and increase your risk of osteoporosis, according to a 2008 study involving 2,500 women. Fizzy drinks contain high levels of phosphoric acid, which leaches calcium from the bones. Researchers at Tufts University in the US recommend sticking to no more than two drinks per week.

Daily calcium requirement (mg)

4–6 years (boys and girls)	450
7–10 years (boys and girls)	550
11–18 years (boys)	1,000
11–18 years (girls)	800
18+ years	700
During pregnancy	no extra
While breast-feeding	550 extra

Foods containing 200mg calcium

Milk	1 glass (170ml)
Milkshake	1 glass (180ml)
Cheddar cheese	1 slice (25g)
Yoghurt	1 carton (130g)
Broccoli	10 sprigs (500g)
Oranges	3 oranges
Sesame seeds	2tbsp (30g)
Tinned sardines	1½ (36g)
Almonds	50 nuts (83g)
Dried figs	4 figs (80g)
Pizza	1 slice (105g)
Tofu	1 slice (40g)
Ice cream	2½ scoops (250g)

Will calcium pills stop me getting osteoporosis?

A study in the *Lancet* gathered all the evidence on bone density and fracture risk and found that calcium or calcium plus vitamin D reduced fracture risk by 12 per cent in people over fifty and reduced bone loss in the hip by 46 per cent. But a 2008 trial involving 1,500 women in New Zealand found that those taking calcium pills had double the risk of heart attack.

Reasons to eat more fruit and vegetables

Research at the MRC Human Nutrition Research in Cambridge, UK in 2006 found that people who had the highest intakes of fruit and vegetables had a higher bone density. It may be due to the vitamin C or potassium content or other fruit-specific antioxidants, or a reduction in the production of acidity in the body with diets rich in fruit and vegetables. When you eat too much acidic food (animal proteins) your body draws on the alkaline calcium in your bones to counteract the acidity. Because fruit and vegetables are alkaline they do not cause the bones to release calcium.

Can osteoporosis be treated?

Once you've lost bone mass, it can't be regained, but you can prevent further damage by strengthening the remaining bone structure and preventing further thinning. Medication may include calcium and vitamin D supplements, hormone treatment, including HRT, and bisphosphonates (drugs that prevent bone breakdown).

Resources

The following organisations are useful if you want to find out more information about any of the topics covered in this book.

American Dietetic Association www.eatright.org
  Nutrition news, tips and resources.

Beat/the Eating Disorders Association www.b-eat.com
  Information and help on all aspects of eating disorders.

British Dietetic Association www.bda.uk.com
  Fact sheets and information on healthy eating and details of
  Registered Dietitians working in private practice.

The British Heart Foundation www.bhf.org.uk
  Information on keeping your heart healthy, healthy eating,
  exercise, kids' fitness and preventing heart disease.

British Nutrition Foundation www.nutrition.org.uk
  Information, fact sheets and educational resources on nutrition
  and health.

Diabetes UK www.diabetes.org.uk
  Authoritative information on living with diabetes, as well as
  sections for children, teenagers and young adults.

Ediets www.ediets.com
  Personalised diet plans, as well as health and fitness features,
  recipes and online support.

Food Commission www.foodcomm.org.uk
  Up-to-date news of nutrition campaigns, surveys and the Parents
  Jury.

Food Standards Agency www.eatwell.gov.uk
Information on healthy eating, food labelling, food safety and health issues.

Health Supplements Information Service www.hsis.org
Information on vitamins, minerals and supplements.

H.E.A.R.T. UK www.heartuk.org.uk
Downloadable fact sheets on many aspects of cholesterol and healthy eating, as well as recipes.

The Mayo Clinic www.mayohealth.org
Nutrition and health information in a fun, user-friendly format.

National Osteoporosis Society www.nos.org.uk
Useful advice about osteoporosis, as well as downloadable information sheets on diet, drug treatments, exercise and many related health conditions.

Vegetarian Society www.vegsoc.org
Information on vegetarian nutrition for children as well as general nutrition, health and recipes.

WebMD www.webmd.com
A–Z directory of health topics and advice on many aspects of nutrition and fitness.

Weight Concern www.weightconcern.com
Excellent information on obesity issues, including a section on children's health and a BMI calculator.

Weight Loss Resources www.weightlossresources.co.uk
Excellent information on weight loss, fitness and healthy eating as well as a comprehensive calorie database and a personalised weight loss programme.

World Cancer Research Fund www.wcrf-uk.org
Accessible advice on cancer prevention including information on diet, physical activity and weight control.

Index